AMERICAN HEALTHCARE UNSTAINABLE

Rebuild Before Collapse

RAVINDER NATH BHALLA MD

AMERICAN HEALTHCARE UNSUSTAINABLE: Rebuild Before Collapse

A Note on Patient Confidentiality

All references to clinical encounters in this book are composite portraits drawn from forty years of psychiatric practice and medical directorship. No patient is identifiable. Names, identifying details, and circumstances have been altered to protect confidentiality while preserving the clinical truths the encounters illustrate. Where public figures (Alec Smith, Robert Allen, Trishaun Holland) are named, the accounts are drawn from publicly reported sources cited in the back matter.

A Note on Citation

Statistical figures, policy citations, and named cases are drawn from published research, government data, and journalism cited in the Sources section at the back of this book.

This book is part of the author's body of work, which includes:

The Abundance Series — seven volumes:

ABUNDANCE

The Two Minds: Choosing Abundance Over Scarcity

Red Lines Rising: Time to Constrain Power Before AI Makes It Permanent

Abundance Dispatch

The Constitution: The Floor Missing

Building Abundance

The Abundance Life

Other works:

Wisdom in Psychiatry: Understanding Begins Healing

Nietzsche: A Guided Tour — A Path Through His Works (two-volume box set)

Wealth, Mind and Meaning: The Money Book Nobody Gave You

What Does It Mean to Be Human In the Age of Robots and Augmented Intelligence

The World Constitution: What We Owe to Our Children Present and Future

Before the Birth of Hope and Despair: On Life, Death, and Heritage (forthcoming)

ISBN: 978-1-971562-65-0 Ebook

978-1-971562-66-7 Paperback

978-1-971562-67-4 Hardback

978-1-971562-68-1 Audio

First edition, 2026

Published by the author

ravibhallamd.com

For Alec Smith, dead at twenty-six from insulin he could not afford —
and for every patient I have sat across from who arrived with the courage
the room required, while the system in which we met
was already extracting the cost of their arrival.
The floor was never built.
It is time to build it.

"The goal is not to choose one truth but to understand why both truths exist.
The transformative power of being understood in complexity:
when a patient realizes that they do not need to simplify themselves
to be taken seriously, something fundamental shifts."
— from Wisdom in Psychiatry by the author

ABUNDANCE ORIENTATION: WHAT THIS BOOK MEANS BY IT

The term abundance orientation appears in this book. It does not mean wealth. It does not mean optimism or positive thinking. It is a specific psychological stance toward the world, and it has a clinical meaning.

A person organized around scarcity experiences their resources — time, love, attention, safety, connection — as fundamentally insufficient. The scarcity orientation is not always delusional. For many people, resources were genuinely scarce, often in childhood, often in the environments that shaped them. The problem is that the orientation persists after conditions change. The adult who grew up with real scarcity often carries its psychological architecture into a life where the original conditions no longer apply. The executive with every material resource continues to hoard, compete, and protect as though the next threat is always imminent. The parent who was never held securely struggles to hold their child securely — not from lack of love, but from lack of the internal template.

A person organized around abundance experiences their resources as workable — not unlimited, not without constraint, but sufficient to act from rather than hide behind. The abundance orientation does not deny difficulty or real scarcity. It refuses to let scarcity be the organizing principle of every decision.

This is not a motivational idea. It is a developmental and neurological one. Chronic scarcity — of safety, of reliable connection, of predictability — shapes neural architecture in ways that are measurable and documented. Chronic abundance — not of money but of secure attachment, of good-enough parenting, of environments where the child's needs are reliably met — shapes neural architecture in ways that are equally measurable in the other direction. The clinical observation that connects it is consistent: children who receive what they need do not spend their lives compensating for what they did not get.

This book argues that abundance orientation is not primarily a personal achievement. It is something that conditions either produce or fail to produce. If the conditions that produce abundance orientation are knowable and buildable, then the failure to build them is a choice, and its costs fall on real children. Readers who wish to explore the larger argument will find it in the Abundance Series at ravibhallamd.com.

Acknowledgments

This book exists because forty years of patients sat across from me and trusted me with the truth of what was happening to them, even when the truth was that the system meant to care for them was extracting the cost of their lives. They are the book's deepest source. Every one of them is unnamed, anonymized, and composite. Every one of them is real.

To Elizabeth, clinical director and longtime colleague, whose direct sentences across years of shared work cut through the temptation to soften what needed to be named.

To the medical directors, hospital administrators, and physician colleagues who have stayed inside the broken system because the patients in front of them needed someone to stay. Their continued presence inside institutions that destroy them is the moral evidence the book draws on.

To my severely autistic son, who has taught me — through every clinical encounter, every insurance denial, every fight for the personal care assistance hours he requires — what the constitutional hole looks like when the floor that should have been built was not. He is the reason I know the rebuild is not theoretical.

To the policy researchers, journalists, and physician-writers whose work made the empirical case undeniable, and whose names appear in the Sources section.

And to Claude (Anthropic), whose editorial assistance through the final phases of this manuscript sharpened arguments that needed sharpening and tested arguments that needed testing. The depth came from the human. The collaboration was real.

Contents

Preface

I HAVE SAT ACROSS FROM BOTH SIDES OF THIS

I want to begin with three rooms.

The first room is the consulting room. Forty years of it. The person across from me has already done something before they arrived — they have simplified themselves. They have taken the complexity of what is happening to them and translated it into what they believe the system can receive. Symptoms. A timeline. A list. They have done this because every institution they have encountered on the way to this room has rewarded the simplified version and penalized the full one. The insurance form wants a diagnosis code. The referral letter wants a chief complaint. The intake coordinator wants to know if they are a danger to themselves or others. By the time they sit down across from me they have learned, efficiently and without being taught explicitly, that the system is not built for the whole person. It is built for the presentation.

The second room is the medical director's office. Thirty-four years of it. I served as medical director of a nonprofit serving three to four thousand people with serious mental illness — people at the bottom of every system the society had built. From that room I watched what happens when the clinical encounter meets the administrative apparatus. I watched a staff that showed up in conditions never adequately resourced and served anyway. I watched prior authorization denials arrive and clinical judgment get subordinated to an insurance algorithm. I watched the billing system consume hours that should have been spent with patients. I watched moral injury develop in real time in people who had entered their professions to heal and were being required, systematically and by design, to do something else.

The third room is the one that cost me the most to understand. I am the father of a severely autistic son who is nonverbal and requires complete care every day of his life. Ten years ago I had to litigate with the Managed Care Organization that administers his PPP — the Personal Preference Program, providing personal care hours funded through Medicaid — which was attempting to reduce his hours. An agreement was reached: hours reduced from forty to thirty-seven, a face-saving win for the MCO. Recently we received another notice. This time the MCO declared that he does not need these services at all. Another litigation is in the making. I am a psychiatrist. I knew the law, the clinical literature, the advocacy landscape. I had colleagues I could call and resources to retain legal representation. It still took litigation. It still took two years. I watched other families navigating identical battles with far less — with no professional knowledge of the system, no network, no ability to absorb the cost of fighting — and I understood something from that room that the consulting room and the medical director's office had not fully taught me: the failures of the American healthcare system are not a matter of individual cases falling through the cracks. The cracks are the system. The falling through is the design.

I have written about this from different angles across my books. About the scarcity orientation — a psychological orientation prophesying scarce resources to be dispensed carefully as a showcase for profitability — that institutions transmit and reproduce. About the body sustained while the person inside it is denied. About the constitutional floor that was never built beneath the patient. About the clinical wisdom that the system suppresses by eliminating the time it requires.

This book holds those arguments together and makes them as one argument, as directly as I know how.

The American healthcare system is unsustainable because it is optimized for the wrong output — and the wrong output is not accidental, it is the direct consequence of treating the patient as a set of symptoms to be processed rather than a person to be cared for, the care encounter as a billable transaction rather than a healing relationship, and the system itself as an extraction apparatus rather than a constitutional floor.

That sentence is the book. Every chapter is the evidence for one of its three clauses.

I am not writing as a policy analyst, though the policy arguments are here and they are documented. I am writing as a psychiatrist who has spent forty years sitting across from what the system produces — the person who has simplified themselves to survive the encounter, the clinician worn down to the point of departure from the work they came to do, the family that won the legal battle and still lost years they cannot recover.

I am also writing because the collapse the title names is not theoretical. It is in progress. One hundred and forty-six rural hospitals closed since 2010. More than half of American physicians report burnout. A man in North Carolina named Alec Smith rationed his insulin because he could not afford three hundred and fifty dollars per vial. He was twenty-six, white, and employed. He died three days after his prescription ran out. The insulin costs between three and ten dollars to manufacture. The gap between three dollars and three hundred and fifty dollars is not a market. It is an apparatus. And the apparatus is not failing. It is functioning exactly as it was built to function — for everyone except the patient at the end of the chain.

A note on what rebuild means

The word *rebuild* in the title is deliberate. Not reform. Not improve. Not fix. Rebuild. Reform assumes the foundation is sound and the structure needs adjustment. The foundation is not sound. The foundation is the constitutional absence of any floor beneath the patient — the legal structure that the government has no affirmative obligation to provide care even when it watches the person deteriorate. Every other wealthy democracy built a floor. We built an extraction apparatus and called it a healthcare system.

Rebuilding means starting with the question no one wants to answer: *who is the healthcare system for?* The answer is the only one that produces a sustainable system. The healthcare system is for the patient. the whole person, the whole one, the one who arrived in the consulting room having already simplified themselves to survive the encounter. Part Two and Part Three of this book make the case for what that means structurally — what a system organized around the right patient looks like, what it costs, and how every other wealthy democracy has already built it.

Somebody decided that Alec Smith's life was worth less than the extraction margin. That decision was made in legislation, in regulatory approval, in campaign finance, in the revolving door between industry and the agencies nominally overseeing it. It was not made once. It has been remade, continuously and deliberately, for decades. It can be made differently. The window for rebuilding before collapse is open. This book is the argument for using it.

A note on the clinical material: all patient accounts are drawn from forty years of practice and are presented in composite, anonymized form. No individual is identifiable from any description in this book. The system failures described are structural, not individual — the clinicians inside them are, in most cases, doing exactly what the people who entered medicine to heal would do inside a system that was not built for healing.

PART I

How It Is Not Working

1

Alec Smith and the Apparatus That Killed Him

Alec Smith, described briefly in the preface, had Type 1 diabetes — not the lifestyle-associated kind, the kind you are born with, the kind that requires insulin every day or you die. The insulin his pharmacy charged three hundred and fifty dollars per vial. He could not afford it. He rationed what he had. He died three days after his prescription ran out. The insulin that killed him by its absence costs between three and ten dollars to manufacture.

The gap between three dollars and three hundred and fifty dollars is not a market inefficiency. It is not a pricing anomaly. It is not the unfortunate byproduct of an otherwise functional system. It is an apparatus — constructed layer by layer over decades, maintained by deliberate political investment, operating exactly as it was built to operate. Alec Smith did not fall through a crack. He fell through a design. He is not an outlier. He is the American healthcare system described from the inside, from the position of the person at the end of the chain.

The political story told about American healthcare — that its failures are primarily a story about race, about the undeserving poor, about urban emergency rooms — is the extraction system's most effective misdirection. The majority of Americans without adequate healthcare, rationing medication, filing for medical bankruptcy, or dying of preventable conditions are white. They are the former plant worker in rural Ohio, the uninsured small business owner in Tennessee, the truck driver who cannot afford the follow-up after the emergency room visit. The extraction system has survived for decades in part by convincing its primary victims that the problem belongs to someone else. Understanding why Alec Smith died requires understanding the apparatus that killed him. It has five layers.

Layer One: The Insurance Company

You pay premiums every month — whether you are sick or not, whether you use the system or not. The insurance company collects that money. When you get sick and need care, the insurance company's financial interest is to pay out as little of it as possible. Every claim it denies is money it keeps. Every procedure it delays through prior authorization is money it holds longer. Every narrow network that steers you away from the specialist you need is a cost it avoids. This is not incidental to the business. It is the business.

The insurance company is legally permitted to profit from the gap between what you pay in and what they pay out for your care. They employ armies of staff whose sole function is to find reasons to deny or delay your claims. Hospitals and doctors employ equally large armies whose sole function is to fight those denials. Thirty cents of every healthcare dollar in the United States is consumed by this war. In Canada, one payer. Administrative costs at twelve cents per dollar. In Taiwan, six cents. The difference — eighteen to twenty-four cents per dollar on a four-and-a-half-trillion-dollar system — is somewhere between eight hundred billion and one trillion dollars every year. Spent not on care. Spent on the machinery of denial.

Layer Two: The Drug Manufacturer

The United States is the only wealthy nation on earth that does not negotiate drug prices. Medicare — the largest single drug purchaser in the world — was legally prohibited from negotiating prices until 2022, and the prohibition that remains covers the vast majority of drugs. That prohibition was written into law in 2003 by pharmaceutical industry lobbyists. Congress passed it. Humira, the best-selling drug in American history, costs around seventy-seven thousand dollars per year in the United States. In Germany: eight thousand dollars. Same drug. Same company. Same molecule. The difference is the absence of negotiation — by legal design, written by the industry that benefits from its absence.

Insulin was discovered in 1921. The inventors sold the patent to the University of Toronto for one dollar each, explicitly so that it could be made available to everyone who needed it. One hundred years later, a man in North Carolina died because he could not afford it.

Layer Three: The Pharmacy Benefit Manager

Pharmacy benefit managers — PBMs — sit between the drug manufacturer and the pharmacy. Their stated purpose is to negotiate discounts on drugs for insurers and employers. What they actually do: demand rebates from drug manufacturers, keep the rebates rather than passing them to the patient, charge the insurer more than they pay the pharmacy, and steer patients toward expensive branded drugs because the rebate on the branded drug is larger.

Mark Cuban's Cost Plus Drugs made the mechanism undeniable. He bypassed the PBM entirely and sold generic drugs at manufacturing cost plus fifteen percent, openly published. A drug that cost three hundred and fifty dollars at a standard pharmacy cost eight dollars at Cost Plus. The PBM was not adding value. It was extracting three hundred and forty-two dollars from every patient who needed that drug, invisibly, where no one was required to disclose what was happening.

Layer Four: The Hospital

Hospitals have merged at a rapid pace over the past three decades. The Federal Trade Commission has documented consistently: hospital mergers raise prices fifteen to forty percent without improving quality or access. Inside every hospital is a chargemaster — an internal price list with no relationship to actual cost. A Tylenol tablet at sixty dollars. A bag of saline at a thousand. An appendectomy at eighty thousand dollars that costs twelve thousand in Germany. The chargemaster exists to set an inflated starting price from which negotiated discounts are calculated — leaving insured patients paying inflated negotiated rates, and uninsured patients, with no negotiating power, facing the full fiction. Approximately one in six emergency room patients without insurance will file for bankruptcy after the visit.

Layer Five: The Revolving Door

Each of the four layers above should have been regulated or dismantled long ago. The evidence for their harm has been available for decades. The officials who are supposed to regulate the pharmaceutical industry frequently come from the pharmaceutical industry and return to it after government service. The congressional staff members who write healthcare legislation frequently move to industry lobbying positions when their tenure ends. The healthcare industry spends more on federal lobbying than any other sector in the American economy. In the 2020 election cycle, pharmaceutical and health products companies alone spent over three hundred million dollars. The return on that investment — measured in preserved drug pricing power, defeated public option proposals, maintained PBM opacity — runs to the trillions.

Following one patient through the chain

Robert is fifty years old. He lives in rural Kentucky. He works. He is insured through his employer. He has Type 2 diabetes and high blood pressure. He pays six hundred dollars a month in insurance premiums. His employer pays another eight hundred on his behalf. Twenty thousand four hundred dollars a year — before Robert has received a single minute of care.

His doctor prescribes a GLP-1 medication that has shown remarkable results for both diabetes management and cardiovascular protection. It costs approximately a thousand dollars per month in the United States. In Canada: two hundred dollars. In Germany: one hundred and eighty dollars. Robert's insurance requires prior authorization. The authorization is denied on the first submission. After appeal, six weeks later, it is approved. Robert has been managing without the medication for six weeks. His blood sugar during that period has caused additional vascular damage that will not be visible for another five years. It will express itself as a hospitalization at a cost of tens of thousands of dollars — recorded as a new medical expense, untethered in any accounting from the six-week delay that contributed to it.

Robert is not a victim of a broken system. He is the product of a functional one — functional for the insurance company, the PBM, the drug manufacturer, the hospital system, and the lobbyists who maintain the apparatus. In Germany, Robert's out-of-pocket exposure would be capped at two percent of his annual income. His emergency room visit would generate no bill at all. The difference between Robert in Kentucky and Robert in Germany is not medical science or technology. It is the decision about who the healthcare system is for. One country decided it is for the patient. The other decided it is for the chain.

Who decided

The opioid epidemic is the extraction system's most complete and catastrophic product. Purdue Pharma marketed OxyContin to physicians across working-class white America with documented misrepresentation of its addiction potential. The FDA approved it. The DEA failed to regulate its distribution. The physicians who prescribed it were operating inside a system that reimbursed procedures and prescriptions but not the time-intensive work of addiction prevention and treatment. The communities saturated with opioids were predominantly white, rural, and working class — the same communities that had lost manufacturing employment, whose mental health infrastructure had been cut, whose political representatives had spent decades opposing the healthcare expansion that might have funded treatment. Eight hundred thousand Americans died of opioid overdose between 1999 and 2022.

The question the extraction system cannot answer is the one the nine-year-old in Chicago asked: *I don't think that is just how it is. I think somebody decided that is how it is.* She is right. Somebody decided. Across decades, in legislation written by lobbyists, in regulatory approvals made by officials who would later work for the industries they regulated — somebody decided that the extraction margin was worth more than Alec Smith's life. The next two chapters explain what the system does to the people inside it and why those decisions have not been reversed. Then the book turns to the deeper question: what kind of system produces these decisions in the first place, and why does the person inside it — patient, clinician, administrator — keep experiencing something that does not feel like care?

2

What the System Does to the People Inside It

There is a particular expression that appears on the face of a physician who has been practicing for ten years or more inside the American healthcare system. It is not exhaustion exactly, though exhaustion is part of it. It is something more specific — the expression of a person who entered their work with a clear sense of purpose and has been required, daily and by design, to act in ways that violate it. Moral injury is the clinical term. It was coined in a military context — the damage done to soldiers required to participate in actions that violated their moral code — and it applies with equal precision to the physician who entered medicine to heal and spends her afternoon on the phone with an insurance company's prior authorization line, explaining to a non-physician reviewer why the medication she prescribed is medically necessary.

She already explained it in the prescription. The reviewer already has the clinical notes. The algorithm has already generated the denial. The call is not a clinical conversation. It is the extraction apparatus consuming forty-five minutes of her time — time that will not appear on any financial statement as a cost of the prior authorization process, because the system has externalized that cost onto the physician's practice the same way it externalizes every other cost it can. She will do this three more times today.

What moral injury is and is not

Moral injury is not burnout. Burnout is the depletion that follows from sustained overwork — treatable with rest, with the restoration of sustainable conditions. Moral injury is different in kind. It is the damage done when a person is required, by the system they operate within, to act in ways that contradict the values that brought them to their work. Burnout depletes. Moral injury corrupts — it damages the person's relationship to their own purpose, their own competence, their own sense of what the work is for. The physician who is burned out needs rest. The physician experiencing moral injury needs the system to stop requiring her to be complicit in the harm of her patients.

More than half of American physicians now report symptoms consistent with burnout — but the term undersells the problem. The leading cause, documented consistently across specialty and practice setting, is not the volume of patients or the complexity of the medicine. It is the administrative burden. The prior authorization. The documentation requirements designed not to capture clinical information but to satisfy the billing apparatus. The electronic health record built for revenue cycle management rather than clinical care. The two hours of administrative work for every one hour of direct patient care.

What it looks like from the inside

I am a psychiatrist and have managed my own sleep apnea with a CPAP machine for more than a decade. The treatment works. My physician knows it works. Fourteen years of continuous CPAP use is the documentation that it works.

In a recent year my insurance plan required a new sleep study before it would authorize a GLP-1 medication for weight management. Not because my condition had changed. Not because the clinical evidence was in question. Because the plan's prior authorization algorithm required a sleep study conducted within the last two years, and mine was fourteen years old.

The sleep study I have not had in fourteen years is not missing because I neglected my health. It is missing because the nonprofit where I served as medical director for thirty-four years had to renegotiate its employee health insurance every few years to survive financially. With each renegotiation, networks changed. My sleep specialist went out of network. I managed my condition with what was available — I purchased my own CPAP machine at one-third of the price I had paid through insurance a decade earlier, navigating the system the way every resourceful patient learns to navigate it. The sleep study was eventually done. It was positive. The medication was approved after a two-month wait. The new CPAP machine prescribed by my sleep doctor has not arrived weeks after the prescription was written.

I have the clinical knowledge, the professional networks, and the language to navigate the system. Most patients do not. Before the sleep study and approval of medication, I sat across from my primary care physician — a young mother of two, already carrying the weight of a practice full of patients navigating similar denials — and I watched, in the set of her face, the expression I described at the beginning of this chapter. She entered medicine to care for patients. She was spending her afternoon managing the bureaucratic consequence of an insurance apparatus designed to exhaust the people inside it until they give up. For the patient without clinical knowledge or professional networks, the exhaustion is the point.

The nursing crisis

Nursing has reached a parallel and in some ways more acute crisis. Nurses are leaving the profession at rates that threaten the basic functioning of the hospital system. The primary reasons documented in exit interviews are not compensation. The reasons are conditions. Understaffing that makes safe care impossible. Administrative demands that displace patient care. Moral injury from being required to provide care that falls below the standard they were trained to meet because the system will not fund the staffing that adequate care requires.

The hospital that runs nursing floors at ratios documented to produce adverse patient outcomes is not making a clinical decision. It is making a financial one. The patient who suffers a preventable complication from understaffing is an externalized cost — appearing as a new diagnosis in a new chart, treated as a new clinical event, billed as a new encounter. The connection between the staffing decision and the adverse outcome is invisible to the financial accounting. So the staffing decision continues.

The rural collapse

One hundred and forty-six rural hospitals have closed in the United States since 2010. Over a thousand more are at financial risk. They are not institutions that failed their communities. They are institutions that served their communities and were destroyed by the financial apparatus of the system they operated within. They are disproportionately dependent on Medicare and Medicaid reimbursement, which is set below the actual cost of care — a structural subsidy extraction that works in urban markets where commercial insurance volume compensates, and fails in rural markets where it does not.

When the hospital closes, what goes with it is not only emergency care. It is the primary care relationships that catch the non-adherence before the hospitalization, the obstetric services that prevent maternal mortality, the mental health beds that interrupt the psychiatric crisis before it cascades. The maternal mortality rate in rural America — disproportionately white, working class — is among the highest in the developed world and is rising. Not because clinical knowledge has declined. Because the obstetric unit is now forty-five minutes away. For a postpartum hemorrhage, that is the difference between life and death.

What wisdom the system suppresses

There is a dimension of the system's damage that the financial analysis does not capture. The American healthcare system suppresses clinical wisdom. Not deliberately — the system has no interest in clinical wisdom one way or another. But the apparatus that eliminates time eliminates the conditions under which clinical wisdom operates.

Wisdom in clinical practice is not the same as knowledge. Knowledge is the diagnostic criteria, the treatment algorithm, the evidence-based protocol. Wisdom is what accumulates across thousands of encounters — the capacity to hear what is behind what is being said, to notice the discrepancy between the symptom reported and the distress communicated, to understand that the patient who presents with low energy and fog may be grieving the music he abandoned rather than manifesting depression, to recognize that dropout from treatment is often the psyche protecting itself rather than the patient failing the treatment. That capacity requires genuine attention, unhurried presence, the willingness to follow the thread that leads away from the chief complaint into the reality of the person's life that produced it. The fifteen-minute appointment slot trains the clinician to receive the presentation rather than the person.

The nonprofit at the edge of the cliff

For forty years I served as medical director of a psychiatric nonprofit serving three to four thousand people with serious mental illness — people at the bottom of every system the society had built. The reimbursement rates set by the state and the insurance plans that contracted with us were reduced every year, consistently below the actual cost of the care we provided. Staff were paid below market rates for their positions. They came to work knowing that the work they had been trained to do could not be fully done within the resources they had been given. They did it anyway.

That commitment is the abundance orientation — a psychological orientation of giving, accepting the conditions, and proceeding to do the right thing — operating inside the scarcity system. It is what the extraction apparatus runs on: the moral reserves of the people inside it, the gap between what is reimbursed and what is required, filled every day by clinical staff who have not yet been fully worn down. Those reserves are finite. I watched them deplete across three and a half decades. The suffering I witnessed was not necessary. That is the conviction on which every argument in this book stands. The system is consuming its own clinical capital. The knowledge can be replaced. The wisdom cannot be replaced on any timeline the system recognizes. The window for rebuild is the window before the people who still hold that wisdom are gone.

3

Why It Does Not Change

The question is not complicated to ask. Majorities of Americans have supported universal healthcare coverage, drug price negotiation, and insurance regulation in every poll taken on the subject for more than two decades. The outcomes of the current system are documented, widely published, and not in serious scientific dispute. The alternatives — demonstrated in every other wealthy democracy — produce better outcomes at lower cost. The people inside the system, patients and clinicians alike, are being destroyed by it. Why does it not change?

The easy answer is corruption. It is not wrong, but it is incomplete — and its incompleteness is itself part of how the system survives. The mechanism is more structural, more legal, more invisible, and more durable. It operates not through individual venality but through the systematic alignment of institutional interests with political outcomes, maintained by a campaign financing apparatus that the Supreme Court has ruled cannot be limited.

The campaign financing apparatus

The healthcare industry spends more on federal lobbying than any other sector in the American economy. In the 2020 election cycle, pharmaceutical and health products companies alone spent over three hundred million dollars on lobbying and campaign contributions. This expenditure is not primarily aimed at changing public opinion — public opinion is already against the industry on every major question. It is aimed at something more specific: the individual legislators on the individual committees that write the individual bills governing pharmaceutical pricing, insurance regulation, and hospital consolidation review.

A senator on the Finance Committee who receives substantial pharmaceutical industry donations does not need to oppose drug price negotiation publicly. She needs only to ensure that the bill that reaches the floor has been amended to protect the pricing apparatus — or that the bill does not reach the floor at all. The amendment happens in committee. The non-scheduling happens in the majority leader's office. Neither event is reported as a vote. The senator's public position remains consistent with her constituents' preferences. The legislation that would change the system never arrives. This is not corruption in the legal sense. Every dollar was reported. Every relationship was disclosed. The Supreme Court in Citizens United ruled that corporate political expenditures are protected speech and cannot be limited. The return on the three hundred million dollar investment runs to the trillions. It is the most efficient capital allocation in American business.

The revolving door

The official who approves a drug at the FDA becomes the lobbyist for the manufacturer. The congressional staff member who writes the Medicare prescription drug benefit joins the pharmaceutical industry trade association. The insurance company executive becomes the state insurance commissioner. These are the documented operational patterns of every major healthcare regulatory agency in the federal government. The revolving door produces regulatory capture — not through conspiracy but through the systematic alignment of institutional perspective with institutional interest. The regulator who came from industry, who will return to industry, who talks daily with industry representatives and rarely with patients — that regulator sees the world through a different lens. The lens was ground by the industry.

The psychology of misdirection

The campaign financing apparatus and the revolving door explain why the system is politically immune to majority preference. They do not fully explain why the majority does not respond with greater political force. For that we need to understand the third mechanism: the systematic misdirection that has kept the system's primary victims from recognizing their common interest.

The American healthcare crisis is primarily a crisis of the white working class. The majority of Americans without adequate healthcare, rationing medication, filing for medical bankruptcy, losing family members to opioid overdose, watching their county hospital close — are white, working class, and living outside major cities. The political story told about American healthcare has been constructed, deliberately and with considerable sophistication, to obscure this fact. The narrative that healthcare reform primarily benefits urban minorities, that the Affordable Care Act was a transfer from the working class to the undeserving poor, that universal coverage is socialism — these narratives were produced and distributed by the industries that benefit from the status quo, through the media infrastructure those industries substantially fund, to the audiences most threatened by the system and most strategically misdirected about who their allies are.

Consider a composite figure who stands in for many thousands of real ones. He is fifty-three years old, white, a former manufacturing worker in rural West Virginia whose plant closed in 2018. He voted against the Affordable Care Act and against Medicaid expansion because he was told, persuasively and repeatedly, that these programs primarily helped people who had not worked as hard as he had. He was uninsured for two years after the plant closed. His wife developed a thyroid condition during that period that went undiagnosed because they could not afford the appointment. When he found work again he waited ninety days for coverage to begin. During those ninety days his wife's untreated condition progressed. The thyroid medication she eventually needed cost forty dollars a month through the new insurance plan — after a prior authorization process that took six weeks and required three phone calls he made from the parking lot of the plant during his lunch break, because he could not make personal calls on the floor. He is grateful for the coverage. He experiences it as earned. He does not connect the thyroid progression to the ninety-day wait or the six-week prior authorization, because the system has never connected those dots for him. He would vote the same way again. The system that harmed him has also given him the framework for understanding the harm.

The scarcity system reproduces itself

There is a fourth mechanism that operates beneath the three structural ones — and it is the one that policy analysis cannot reach but clinical analysis can. The scarcity orientation is not only individual. It is institutional. It transmits from institution to institution through the reward structures that reinforce it, the selection mechanisms that promote the people who embody it, and the systematic exclusion of the orientation that would challenge it.

The insurance company reviewer who denies the prior authorization is executing an algorithm designed by people trained, selected, and promoted within an institution whose financial model rewards the denial. The hospital administrator who approves the understaffing ratio is operating within a financial model that makes adequate staffing incompatible with the margin required. The pharmaceutical executive who prices insulin at three hundred and fifty dollars is calculating the return on investment his shareholders require. None of these people are villains in the individual sense. They are the output of institutions organized around scarcity — around the question of how to keep as much of the premium as possible — rather than around the question the healthcare system should be organized around: what does this patient need?

Why reform has failed when it has been tried

The Clinton healthcare plan of 1993 was defeated by the Harry and Louise advertising campaign — produced by the Health Insurance Association of America at a cost of approximately twenty million dollars — that successfully repositioned universal coverage as a threat to the coverage Americans already had. It moved public opinion ten points in eight months. The Affordable Care Act of

2010 passed after the insurance industry extracted the individual mandate. The public option was removed before the bill reached the floor. The pharmaceutical industry extracted a prohibition on Medicare negotiation as the price of its neutrality. The ACA's coverage expansion was genuine and consequential — it is not nothing. But it is the favor rather than the floor — coverage extended as a policy, revocable by the next administration, built on a foundation the Supreme Court partially dismantled in NFIB v. Sebelius by making Medicaid expansion optional for states. The states that refused expansion are disproportionately the states with the highest rates of uninsured working-class white populations.

How the system taught its victims to defend it

The most insidious feature of the extraction apparatus is not that it harms the most vulnerable. It is that it has convinced the most vulnerable that the harm is their fault — and that the structural alternative being offered to them is an attack on the very identity the system built for them while it was extracting from them.

The patient with serious mental illness who cycles through hospitalizations — each one documented as a new clinical event, each one treated as the product of the illness rather than the product of the gap between what the illness requires and what the system provides — often believes, because the system has taught them to believe, that the cycling is their failure. The non-adherence is their weakness. The system that produces the cycle has also produced the explanation for the cycle that removes itself from the causal chain. The working-class patient who cannot afford the follow-up appointment, who manages the chronic condition inconsistently because consistent management requires resources the system has not provided, who develops the complication that brings them back to the emergency room — that patient is told, at each encounter, about the importance of medication adherence, dietary compliance, and regular follow-up. The message is delivered sincerely by a clinician who genuinely cares. But the message is: your health outcomes are primarily a function of your choices. The structural conditions that make those choices impossible are invisible to the encounter. The patient leaves having been treated — and having been, once again, taught that the problem is them.

This is how the system permeates. Not through dramatic harm that announces itself as harm. Through the ordinary texture of working life — the ninety-day wait, the prior authorization, the weeks between the prescription and the device — in which each obstacle is navigable, each navigation feels like agency, and the aggregate cost of all of it is diffuse enough to be invisible as a system. The person who knows the system best, who has navigated it longest, who has the clinical expertise and the professional network and still waits weeks for a prescribed device that their doctor ordered — that person is the system's clearest witness. If it does this to the person who understands exactly what it is doing, what does it do to the person who does not?

The self-defeating machine

The American healthcare system has achieved something remarkable: it has made itself maximally expensive by refusing to spend money at the only points where spending is cheap.

It invests nothing in prevention because prevention is not billable. The food desert, the adverse childhood experience, the untreated early depression, the prediabetes that could have been reversed — none of this is the system's problem until it becomes the system's most expensive problem. It delays treatment because delay is financially rational for the entity bearing the current cost but not the future one. The prior authorization that takes six weeks, the ninety-day waiting period, the GLP-1 medication denied until the diabetes is advanced enough that denial becomes harder to defend — each delay is a cost saving recorded in one column and a complication produced in another column that no accounting connects to it.

It then produces complications that were entirely predictable. The vascular damage accumulating during the authorization delay. The wound that will not heal because the diabetes was never adequately controlled. The psychiatric hospitalization that follows the missed follow-up. The overdose that follows the untreated addiction. Each one recorded as a new clinical event. None traceable in any accounting to the upstream decision not to prevent or treat them.

Then it mobilizes an enormous expensive apparatus to contain the cost of the complications its own decisions produced. Prior authorization review. Utilization management. Disease management programs. Discharge planning. Readmission prevention teams. The system that would not spend forty-five dollars a month on the statin spends forty thousand on the cardiac event, then spends additional resources trying to prevent the next one. It is a machine that creates the problem, delays the solution, produces the crisis, pays for the crisis at maximum cost, then exhausts itself managing the consequences — while calling this healthcare.

Every other wealthy healthcare system understands the arithmetic. Prevention is investment. Early treatment is cheaper than late treatment. The complication costs more than the medication that would have prevented it. The hospitalization costs more than the follow-up calls that would have caught the deterioration. This is not complex medicine. It is the arithmetic that every other system has built into its apparatus — and that the American system has systematically excluded, because the entity that would make the upstream investment is never the entity that captures the downstream return.

A system that will not spend a dollar to prevent the disease, delays the treatment until the disease is too advanced to ignore, produces the complication it could have prevented, then exhausts itself managing the cost of the complication it produced — that system is not failing. It is succeeding at the wrong thing. And it will keep succeeding at the wrong thing until somebody decides that the patient at the end of the chain is who the system is for.

PART II

Why It Is Wrong Before It Is Expensive

4

The Person Behind the Presentation

Every patient who enters the American healthcare system has already done something before they arrive. They have edited themselves.

Not consciously, not all at once, but through accumulated experience of what the system can receive and what it cannot. The insurance form wants a diagnosis code. The referral letter wants a chief complaint. The emergency room triage nurse wants to know the primary symptom. The specialist's intake form wants the medications, the allergies, the previous procedures. Every institutional encounter has trained the patient to present themselves as a set of processable data — and to leave behind the parts of themselves that the processing cannot handle.

By the time they sit across from a clinician, they have been processed so many times that the edited version has become, in the clinical encounter, the presenting version. The complexity is still there — the grief, the fear, the work situation that is making the insomnia worse, the family history that makes the diagnosis carry different weight, the cultural context that shapes what the symptom means and what the treatment will require. But none of it arrives unless the clinician creates the conditions that make it possible. And the fifteen-minute appointment slot, the documentation burden, the prior authorization waiting on the computer screen, the seven other patients in the waiting room — none of these create those conditions.

The system was built to receive a presentation. It was not built to receive a person.

Symptoms describe how. Not why.

Symptoms describe how a person suffers. They do not describe why. The diagnostic category captures the presentation. It does not capture the biography that produced it, the meaning the person has made of it, or the conditions of their life that will determine whether treatment succeeds or fails.

A young man comes in with low energy, cognitive fog, and loss of motivation. He meets criteria for major depressive disorder. The system is equipped to respond to that diagnosis: medication options, a referral for therapy, a follow-up in four weeks. What the system is not equipped to ask — and what the fifteen-minute appointment slot does not permit asking — is what was happening in his life eighteen months ago when the symptoms began. In this case: he was a musician who had practiced his instrument daily since childhood, who had been told by the people closest to him that the music was a distraction from his real life, and who had gradually, without making a conscious decision, stopped playing. His symptoms were not a disorder. They were grief wearing a clinical mask. Grief for the abandoned self. The antidepressant would have addressed the mask. Nothing in the encounter was designed to see what was underneath it.

This is not a rare case. It is the ordinary case of clinical practice, multiplied across every specialty and every waiting room. The diabetic patient whose non-adherence to medication is not carelessness but the behavioral expression of a depression that was never diagnosed. The hypertensive patient whose blood pressure does not respond to medication because the stressor producing it is a housing situation that no prescription can address. The child with behavioral problems in school whose presentation resolves when the domestic violence at home is identified and interrupted. The symptom is real.

It is also a message from the whole person about conditions in their life that the biological treatment cannot reach.

The dropout the system calls non-compliance

One of the most consequential — and most misread — clinical phenomena in American healthcare is what the system records as treatment dropout and non-compliance. The patient who stops taking the medication. Who misses the follow-up appointments. Who disengages from treatment after initial engagement. The system records this as the patient's failure. It is very often something else.

In forty years of clinical practice, I have found that dropout from psychiatric treatment frequently represents the psyche doing something intelligent. Premature illumination — the truth arriving faster than the person can metabolize it, the therapeutic process moving toward territory the patient is not yet equipped to enter — produces a self-protective withdrawal that looks like resistance. The patient who abruptly stops coming after several sessions of apparent engagement is often the patient who has begun to feel something that the rest of their life is not yet structured to hold. The dropout is the circuit breaker. It is not failure. It is the psyche's timing, protecting the person from the destabilization that insight without support produces.

The system that records this as non-compliance and closes the file has misread the clinical data. The appropriate response is to create the conditions — the slower pace, the explicit naming of what feels threatening about the process, the adjustment of the treatment relationship to what the patient can currently use — that make re-engagement possible on the patient's terms rather than the system's schedule. This requires the time, the relational continuity, and the clinical wisdom that the fifteen-minute appointment slot and the high-turnover staffing model systematically eliminate.

Non-compliance with medication in chronic disease follows the same pattern. The diabetic patient who stops taking insulin regularly is not indifferent to their health. They are managing something the medication schedule has failed to account for — the cost, the side effects that were not adequately explained, the dosing complexity that conflicts with a work schedule the prescribing physician did not ask about, the cultural significance of the dietary changes required, the depression that makes all self-care difficult and that nobody has addressed. Non-adherence is clinical information. The system treats it as patient failure.

What understanding in complexity produces

The epigraph of this book comes from *Wisdom in Psychiatry*: *When a patient realizes that they do not need to simplify themselves to be taken seriously, something fundamental shifts.* That shift is not a philosophical preference or a luxury of more leisurely clinical practice. It is the mechanism of healing in every domain where the whole person determines the outcome. And in chronic disease, in mental illness, in substance use disorders, in the conditions that drive the highest costs in the American healthcare system — the whole person determines the outcome almost entirely.

The patient who is understood in complexity becomes a different participant in their own care. They bring more information. They report symptoms more accurately because they have stopped filtering for what they think the system wants to hear. They engage with treatment differently because the treatment has been designed around their actual life rather than around the diagnostic category that fits their presentation. The therapeutic relationship — the specific experience of being seen by another person and not found wanting — is itself a clinical intervention, with documented effects on treatment adherence, symptom reduction, and long-term functioning.

None of this appears in a billing code. The insurance company has no reimbursement category for *patient experienced sufficient relational safety to disclose the actual cause of their symptoms.* The outcome — avoided hospitalization, avoided medication escalation, avoided the crisis that the unaddressed biographical condition would eventually have produced — is invisible to the financial accounting. The cost of not having that conversation will appear years later as a new clinical event, untethered in any accounting from the conversation that never happened.

the whole person and the extraction apparatus

The extraction apparatus and the failure to see the whole person are not separate problems. They are the same problem expressed at different scales. The billing code that cannot capture the conversation that would have prevented the crisis is the financial expression of the same architectural blindness that built a system around the presenting symptoms and left the whole person out.

The physician who has two hours of administrative work for every hour of clinical care has not merely lost time. They have lost the conditions under which the whole person becomes visible. The fifteen-minute appointment slot is not only a scheduling constraint. It is a clinical constraint — it determines what can be received, what can be asked, what can be understood. The electronic health record optimized for billing rather than clinical thinking is not only an administrative burden. It is a cognitive apparatus that trains the clinician to see the patient as a series of fields to be completed rather than a person to be understood.

The system that cannot see the whole person cannot treat the whole person. And the diseases that are destroying the system's financial sustainability — the chronic conditions, the mental health crises, the substance use disorders, the non-healing wounds, the cycling hospitalizations — are primarily diseases of the whole person. They are conditions whose trajectory is determined by the conditions of a life, by the history that produced the presentation, by the meaning the person makes of what is happening to them and what the treatment requires. You cannot treat them with the presenting symptoms alone. You can only manage the biological consequences of the conditions of the person's life you have chosen not to address. And managing those consequences indefinitely is what unsustainable looks like.

What this means for the rebuild

The rebuild this book argues for in Part Three is not primarily a financial restructuring, though the financial restructuring is necessary. It is a clinical one: redesign the system to receive the person rather than the presentation. This requires time — which requires staffing ratios that make time possible, which requires a payment apparatus that funds time rather than only for procedures. It requires relational continuity — the patient who sees the same clinician across multiple encounters, who does not have to re-edit themselves for a new provider each time, who can build the kind of clinical relationship in which the whole person eventually becomes visible. It requires clinical wisdom — the accumulated capacity to hear what is behind what is being said, which is not teachable in a medical school curriculum and not preservable in a system that eliminates the conditions under which it develops.

Most fundamentally it requires the recognition that the most expensive patient in the American healthcare system is not the one with the most severe disease at the moment of presentation. It is the one whose the conditions of the person's life were never addressed, whose non-adherence was never understood, whose dropout was never correctly read, whose symptom was treated and whose life was not. That patient returns. They always return. And each return is more expensive than the conversation that would have prevented it.

The system built to receive the presentation will keep paying for the person it refused to see.

5

The Body Is Not the Patient

There is a thought that every parent of a child with severe disability has had. It comes in a moment of exhaustion or grief or both, and it is so frightening that most people bury it immediately and never speak it aloud. It is the thought that asks whether the life being sustained is the life that was wanted — for the child, not for the parent. Whether the extraordinary measures being deployed are serving the person inside the body or only the body itself. Whether the love that drives the effort to keep the child alive is the same love that would, if it could, release them from the suffering the effort produces.

I have had that thought. I am a psychiatrist. I know its clinical name and its psychological function and the research literature on its prevalence among parents in my situation. I know it does not make me a bad father. I know it is the thought of a person who loves his son enough to look at the full reality of what his son's life contains, rather than the sanitized version that makes the continuing effort feel unambiguous.

I am writing about it here because it is the entry point to the most important distinction this book makes — the distinction that the American healthcare system is constitutionally incapable of processing, that no billing code captures, that no prior authorization algorithm can evaluate, and that determines, more than any other single variable, whether the care delivered is care in any meaningful sense.

The distinction between the body and the person inside it.

What the body does

The body does what it does. The heart beats. The kidneys filter. The lungs exchange gases. The immune system responds to pathogens. The wound repairs. The blood pressure stabilizes. The glucose level registers within an acceptable range. These are measurable, documentable, codeable. They are what the healthcare system was built to address. The system is genuinely extraordinary at addressing them. The clinical science of maintaining the body has produced achievements that would have seemed miraculous a century ago. A person who would have died of infection in 1920 survives. A person who would have died of a cardiac event in 1970 survives. A premature infant at twenty-four weeks in 1990 survives. These survivals are real. the physical life they preserve is the precondition of everything else. But it is only the precondition. Not the thing itself.

What the life behind the presentation is

the life behind the presentation is the life that has a self inside it. The life in which there is a person who has preferences — who wants certain things and does not want others, whose preferences can be expressed and recognized and respected. The life in which there is a history — events that happened to this person, relationships that formed them, losses that changed them, meanings they have made from their experience. The life in which there is a future that can be feared or hoped for, planned toward or prepared for. The life in which the person can say something — about what they need, what they value, what they are willing to endure and what they are not — and be heard.

the person's actual life does not require verbal language. It does not require the capacity for narrative self-reflection or the ability to project a future in words. A person who cannot speak, who cannot construct a linear personal history, who cannot articulate a preference in a form the system recognizes — still has preferences, still experiences comfort and distress, still exists in a web of relational meaning, still has a daily life whose quality is entirely real to the person living it. The actual life of a nonverbal severely disabled person is not lesser than any other. It speaks a language the system was not built to hear.

This is the distinction that matters: not the capacity to narrate, but the existence of a self whose experience has value and whose preferences deserve recognition. Every person who has ever been cared for by another has a full life, regardless of their cognitive or communicative capacity. The system's failure to see it is the system's limitation, not the person's.

The three cases

I have described three patients in an earlier book in this series — their situations drawn from forty years of clinical observation, their details anonymized, their trajectories real. They belong here too, because they are the clinical evidence for the distinction this chapter makes.

The first is a woman in her late nineties. Her physical condition is being maintained with considerable clinical skill — medications optimized, fluid balance managed, skin integrity protected, nutritional needs met. By every medical measure she is receiving excellent care. She is not receiving excellent care. She is receiving excellent physical maintenance. Her the life behind the presentation — her preferences, her history, her sense of what her remaining time should contain — is not visible to the system caring for her. She has expressed, to the family members who visit, a clear preference for a certain kind of ending: in her own space, without extraordinary measures, with the people she loves nearby. This preference is not recorded in her chart in any form that would survive a shift change. The system is doing everything it was built to do. It is not doing what she needs.

The second is a man with diabetes who is losing himself by inches. Not losing his physical capacity — each wound is being addressed, each in turn, with clinical competence. Each wound is cleaned and dressed. Each complication is coded and billed. What is being lost is the person who stood inside all those physical functions and had a life. The system sees the wound. It does not see the person watching himself disappear one limb at a time, or the specific horror of that watching, or what it would require to address that horror as a clinical fact.

The third is my son. He is severely autistic, nonverbal, and requires complete care every day of his life. He arrived with a full life that does not speak the language the system recognizes. He cannot narrate his history or project his future in words. But he has preferences — unmistakable, specific, fully his own. He experiences comfort and joy and fear. He exists in a web of deep relational love. His daily life has a texture that is entirely real to him and entirely visible to the people who know him. The system, however, only sees his physical measurements. It funds his physical survival. It refuses to fund the support required to give that survival dignity and meaning.

The ninety-seven-year-old woman whose peaceful death is denied by an intervention she did not want, the diabetic man whose identity is eroded along with his limbs, and my son whose daily dignity is subject to a prior authorization algorithm — they are all victims of the same systemic blindness. The system treats them as bodies to be managed rather than whole persons to be accompanied. That blindness is not incidental. It is the apparatus.

The grief that has no funeral

I want to say something here about my son that belongs in this argument and cannot be left out. I have written about it at length in a separate book — *Before the Birth of Hope and Despair: On Life, Death, and Heritage* — which addresses what it means to sustain a body while the person living it is not seen, not heard, and not served by the systems nominally caring for them. That book is not a prerequisite for this one. But the experience it describes is the experience that produced this chapter, and the summary that follows is what this argument requires.

There is a kind of loss the culture has no name for. It is not death. It is the presence of someone you love in a form that does not fully return the love — not because the love was withdrawn, but because the capacity to receive and express it in the forms love usually takes was never fully available. You grieve someone who is still in the room. You mourn someone you are also feeding, bathing, advocating for, litigating for. The grief and the caregiving are simultaneous and inseparable, and there is no ceremony for it, no recognized stage, no date after which you are officially mourning.

When Rajeev was two, I watched other children at two. I watched the language arrive — the first words, the sentences, the particular child becoming visible through the talking. It did not arrive. I marked the absence the way you mark the absence of something you were waiting for. Quietly. Without ceremony. When he was five, I watched other children at five. When he was ten. When he was seventeen and other fathers were arguing with their teenage sons and being driven slightly mad by them and also secretly delighted by the people those sons were becoming — I watched that too, from the outside of it. The father I would have been was a presence I kept meeting and losing, at each stage, without anyone to tell me that losing him counted as a loss.

This is the grief that has no funeral. Not the death of the person. The death of the person they might have been — continuous, unstoppable, renewed at every developmental marker that passes without them. You mourn the two-year-old, and then the five-year-old, and then the teenager, and none of these losses has a date or a ritual or a recognized weight. The culture does not have a word for what you are doing. The culture is not watching. You just keep going.

The grief that has no funeral is not only a private matter. It is a public failure. The culture that offers no ritual for this grief, no recognized language for it, no social permission to name what the carrying costs — that culture has decided, by omission, that this grief does not count as grief. As if the presence of the living body resolves the question of what is being mourned. It does not. the life the person is actually living — the self that could have arrived and did not, or that arrived and is being slowly consumed — is absent regardless of what the body is doing. Invisible grief is carried alone, without support, without acknowledgment, in the middle of everything else. Which is the hardest way to carry anything.

Love tested

Almost anyone you share a life with becomes a way. The person you love becomes the shape of your love — not only the object of it but its form, its particular texture, its specific demands and gifts. You do not love someone who has been through what Pascale and I have been through the way you would love someone who has not. The love takes the shape of what it has been asked to hold. And that shape, once formed, becomes who you are.

Rajeev is thirty-four years old. He is gentle. He has a smile that arrives without warning and is entirely his own. He moves through the spaces available to him without demanding more. He does not know what this book is. He carries the oldest thing in us — the primal drive to continue, the survival that stands alone — without the narrative structures the rest of us build around it. To be near him is to be near something that precedes, in evolutionary time, the entire apparatus of meaning-making that the rest of us inhabit. That is not a deficit. It is a different location in the long history of what we are.

The love that goes on regardless — that asks nothing back, receives nothing in the forms love usually requires to sustain itself, and continues — is one of the most demanding things a human being can do. Every parent knows something of this. For a parent like me, the lesson is not softened by an eventual return. It is deepened. What you discover is that the love does not actually need the return in order to be real. It needs only you, continuing to give it. We have this capacity. The carrying costs what it costs. It is also worth what it is worth.

I write about this not to elicit sympathy but because it is the reality of the person's life that the healthcare system I am indicting has never once asked about. In forty years of clinical encounters, in litigation, in prior authorization calls, in fair hearing processes, not one institutional actor has asked what the carrying costs. The system is not built to ask. It is built to process the presenting symptoms. The the reality of the person's life — the grief, the love, the weight in the body of the person who has been doing this work for decades — exists entirely outside the system's field of vision.

The fuller account of what this section describes — the grief, the litigation, the love that has no recognized form — is in *Before the Birth of Hope and Despair* (Bhalla, 2025). The summary offered here is sufficient for this book's argument: the system that cannot see the person cannot see the person caring for them either. Both are invisible to the billing code. Both are real.

The healthcare system breaks down at the boundary between these two kinds of life — not because the clinical knowledge to address the life behind the presentation does not exist, but because the billing apparatus was never built to fund it.

Consider what addressing the whole person actually requires. It requires the conversation in which the clinician asks not only what the patient's blood pressure is but what the patient's life is. It requires the time to hear the answer — not the edited version the patient has learned to present to institutions, but the full version that takes more than fifteen minutes to emerge. It requires the palliative care conversation that happens before the patient is actively dying — the conversation about what this person values, what they are willing to endure, what the best possible version of the remaining time looks like for them rather than for the institution caring for them. It requires the psychiatric consultation that addresses the depression driving the non-adherence, rather than the medication adjustment that addresses the non-adherence as if it were a purely physical phenomenon.

None of this is mysterious. Every clinician who has been in practice for more than a decade knows it. The clinical literature documents it. The outcomes data supports it. The patient who is seen as a whole person — whose treatment is designed around the conditions of their actual life, whose preferences are recorded and respected, whose non-adherence is understood rather than documented as a compliance problem — has better outcomes by every measure the system uses. The system does not fund the conversation. It funds the visit. It funds the procedure. It funds the hospitalization. It funds the code. It does not fund the sustained attention to the whole person that would make the visit and the procedure and the hospitalization either unnecessary or genuinely useful.

Gerry Gelber's observation

A colleague made an observation about my son that has stayed with me for years. He said: if your son had been raised in India, he might not have lived this long. He was not wrong. He was describing a system — or rather the absence of the specific kind of system the United States has built — in which the imperative to sustain the body is less absolute. In which the extraordinary measures are less automatically deployed. In which the question of what the sustained physical life contains for the person living it is asked before the resources of the clinical system are committed to sustaining it.

This observation does not lead where it might appear to lead. It is not an argument for reducing care for people with severe disability. It is an argument about a specific hypocrisy at the center of the American healthcare system that I have experienced personally, documented legally, and watched destroy other families who had fewer resources to survive it.

The American healthcare system will spend millions of dollars in a pediatric intensive care unit to sustain the physical life of a severely disabled child. It will deploy the full apparatus of modern medicine — the ventilators, the specialists, the interventions — without hesitation, without prior authorization delay, without utilization review. The billing codes for physical survival are unambiguous. The system processes them without friction.

Then it will fight the same family in court over three hours of personal care assistance per week.

I know this because it happened to us. Ten years ago I litigated with the Managed Care Organization administering my son's PPP — the Personal Preference Program, which funds personal care hours through Medicaid. The MCO wanted to reduce his hours. After two years of litigation we reached an agreement: hours reduced from forty to thirty-seven. A face-saving win for the MCO. Recently we received another notice. This time the MCO declared that he does not need these services at all. Another litigation is in the making. The system that will not blink at a million-dollar ICU admission is litigating to eliminate the personal care hours that allow a nonverbal man to be bathed, dressed, and taken outside.

That is not a resource allocation problem. It is a values problem. The system values physical survival absolutely and human dignity contingently. It funds the former without question and treats the latter as a discretionary expenditure to be minimized. The result is a system that demands physical survival and abandons the person who lives it. That is the cruelty the Gerry Gelber observation names — not that the American system keeps disabled people alive, but that it insists on the physical survival while systematically starving the life the person is actually living that would give that survival meaning.

The cost of the missing half

The missing half is not only a clinical failure. It is a financial catastrophe at the center of the healthcare system's unsustainability.

The most expensive care in the American healthcare system is care delivered in the last year of life. Approximately a quarter of all Medicare spending occurs in the final year, much of it in the final weeks. The majority of this spending goes to intensive physical interventions — hospitalizations, ICU admissions, procedures, resuscitations — delivered to patients whose the person's preferences, if they had been documented and honored, would not have included these interventions. Study after study has documented the same finding: when patients are asked what they want at the end of life, they consistently describe a version of dying that is less medicalized, less institutionalized, and less expensive than what they typically receive. They want to be home. They want to be comfortable. They want the people they love nearby. They want their preferences to be honored.

They do not get what they want. Not primarily because clinical staff are indifferent to their preferences. Because the system has no mechanism for capturing, documenting, and honoring the person's preferences in the face of the imperative to sustain the body. When the body deteriorates and the clinical system responds with its standard repertoire of interventions, the whole person who would have chosen otherwise is not visible in the chart in any form that survives the urgency of the acute event.

The result is care that is simultaneously more expensive than the patient wanted, less aligned with the patient's values than any clinician would endorse if asked, and clinically less effective at producing the outcome the patient actually defined as a good outcome — because the patient's definition was biographical and the system's is biological.

What the floor requires

The constitutional floor this book argues for — the structural guarantee beneath every patient that the system exists for their benefit rather than for its own perpetuation — must include the whole person. A floor built only on the presenting symptoms is the system we already have. It sustains life without seeing the person who lives it.

The floor that includes the whole person requires four things that the current system systematically withholds. Time — enough clinical time for the conversation in which the whole person becomes visible. Continuity — the relational continuity that makes trust possible, in which the biography accumulates across encounters rather than being re-edited for each new face. Documentation — the recording of the person's preferences in forms that survive shift changes and acute events. And standing — the constitutional standing of the whole person to determine what happens to their body's continued function, honored rather than deferred to the system's convenience.

This applies at every point on the lifespan. Not only at the end of life, where the cost of ignoring it is most immediately visible. At the beginning of life, where the system that sustains the physical survival of a severely disabled infant will then fight the family over the support hours that would give that survival its meaning. In the middle of life, where the diabetic man losing himself limb by limb is receiving excellent biological management and no attention to the whole person. In every room where a patient has simplified themselves to survive the encounter and left the reality of the person's life that is driving the clinical picture at the door.

The three rooms I described in the Preface are three versions of the same failure. The consulting room where the person edits themselves to fit the system's categories. The medical director's office where the bureaucratic apparatus consumes the time that attention to the whole person requires. The family's fight for the care hours that the system will fund a million-dollar ICU to render necessary and then litigate to deny.

The system that sees the presenting symptoms and cannot see the whole person is not providing care. It is providing the performance of care. The rebuild this book argues for begins with the recognition that the person inside the body has always been the patient. The body was only ever the address.

6

The Constitutional Hole

In 1984 a Wisconsin caseworker named Ann Kemmeter began receiving reports that a four-year-old boy named Joshua DeShaney was being beaten by his father. She visited the home. She recorded her observations in her case notes. She noted that Joshua was at risk. She predicted, in writing, that he would be seriously harmed if the situation continued. She did nothing to remove him from the home. She had no legal obligation to do so.

In 1984 Joshua's father beat him so severely that he suffered brain damage leaving him profoundly cognitively impaired for the rest of his life.

His mother sued the Winnebago County Department of Social Services, arguing that the state's failure to protect Joshua from a known threat violated his constitutional rights. In 1989 the Supreme Court of the United States ruled against her. Chief Justice Rehnquist, writing for the majority, held that the Constitution does not require the government to provide services to its citizens, even when the government is aware of a danger to their life. The due process clause is a protection against what the government does to you. It is not a guarantee of what the government will do for you.

The State's failure to protect an individual against private violence does not constitute a violation of the Due Process Clause.

That sentence is the foundation beneath the American healthcare system. Not the Affordable Care Act. Not Medicare. Not any of the policy layers constructed in the decades since. The constitutional bedrock on which everything else either rests or does not is the Supreme Court's holding that the government has no affirmative obligation to protect you from harm, even when it knows the harm is coming, even when it has the capacity to prevent it, even when it has been watching the harm develop and has written down its prediction of the outcome.

The floor was never built. Not because no one tried. Because the constitution, as interpreted by the court, does not require it.

What the constitutional hole means

Every policy built on top of the constitutional hole is built on sand. The Affordable Care Act expanded coverage to millions of Americans. It did so through a combination of Medicaid expansion, premium subsidies, and insurance market regulations. It was a genuine achievement. It is also a policy — enacted by Congress, subject to repeal by Congress, partially dismantled by the Supreme Court in NFIB v. Sebelius when the court made Medicaid expansion optional for states. The states that refused expansion are disproportionately the states with the highest concentrations of the working-class populations the book has been describing.

Medicare is a program. Programs are funded by appropriations. Appropriations are subject to political negotiation. Every year the reimbursement rates that determine whether rural hospitals can remain open, whether psychiatric organizations can staff their clinical programs, whether the primary care physician can afford to run a practice that takes Medicare patients — these rates are set by a political process that the healthcare industry funds and influences through the mechanisms Chapter 3 described.

Medicaid is a matching program. The federal government provides matching funds to states that operate Medicaid programs meeting federal requirements. States can reduce eligibility, restrict benefits, cut reimbursement rates — and they do, regularly, because the political cost of cutting Medicaid falls on populations with the least political power. Programs without constitutional floors are subject to the financial interests of the entities administering them. the life the person is actually living — the personal care hours, the community support, the services that give physical survival its meaning and dignity — is always the first thing cut. Because the constitutional hole sits directly beneath it.

Every one of these programs is real. Every one of them is better than nothing. And every one of them rests on the constitutional hole — on the absence of any structural guarantee that the government must provide healthcare to any person, regardless of their circumstances, regardless of the consequences of its failure to do so. The hole is not hidden. It is the explicit holding of the Supreme Court of the United States, stated clearly in 1989 and confirmed repeatedly since. The civilization built the extraction apparatus on top of it and called it a healthcare system.

What other countries did instead

Germany filled the constitutional hole in 1883. Under Bismarck — not a progressive reformer but a conservative chancellor who understood that a working class without a floor was a working class available for revolution — Germany enacted the world's first statutory health insurance. The logic was not charitable. It was structural: the state that does not provide the floor will eventually pay for the consequences of its absence in ways more expensive and more destabilizing than the floor itself would have cost.

Britain filled it in 1948. In the wreckage of the Second World War, with the political will for structural transformation at its peak, Aneurin Bevan created the National Health Service. The argument was simple: illness is not a personal failing. The treatment of illness is not a market commodity. The healthcare system exists for the patient, and the patient's access to it cannot be contingent on their ability to pay.

Taiwan filled it in 1995. Forty percent uninsured, fragmented private insurance, large gaps for the poor, elderly, and self-employed. Two years of design and implementation. Universal coverage, administrative costs at six percent of total spending, outcomes improving for three consecutive decades. The decision Taiwan made was the same decision Germany and Britain had made: the healthcare system is for the patient, the floor belongs to every person by right of being a person, and the state's obligation to deliver it is not discretionary.

Japan. France. Norway. Australia. Canada. Every wealthy democracy except the United States has made this decision in one form or another. The specific institutional arrangements differ. The underlying constitutional commitment is the same: the state has an affirmative obligation to ensure that no person is denied healthcare because they cannot afford it. The floor exists. The government must maintain it. The United States has not made this decision. Not because the clinical knowledge does not exist. Not because the financial capacity does not exist — the United States spends more on healthcare per capita than any other country on earth while covering fewer people less completely. Because the industries that profit from the constitutional hole have invested, continuously and successfully, in keeping it open.

Justice Brennan's dissent

The DeShaney decision was not unanimous. Justice Brennan, joined by Justices Marshall and Blackmun, dissented. His argument was precise and it has not been answered in the thirty-five years since the decision was handed down.

Brennan wrote that the majority's distinction — between what the state does to you and what the state fails to do for you — was artificial in the specific context of a social services system that had intervened in Joshua's life, created a file, conducted home visits, and made a determination that the risk was present but not sufficient to warrant removal. The state had not simply failed to act in a vacuum. It had acted — incompletely, inadequately, in ways that may have actually reduced the likelihood of private intervention by signaling to neighbors and family members that the situation was being monitored. The state's partial action had created a specific duty that its inaction then violated.

The majority rejected this argument. The constitutional hole remained. But Brennan's dissent is the legal foundation for the floor the rebuild requires — the constitutional recognition that the state which enters a person's life, which creates systems nominally designed to protect them, which takes partial actions that signal to the world that the protection is being provided, has incurred an obligation it cannot discharge by pointing to the negative liberty the majority protected.

The argument of this book is Brennan's argument applied to the healthcare system as a whole. The state has intervened. It has created Medicare and Medicaid and the regulatory apparatus of the insurance market. It has signaled, through those interventions, that the protection is being provided. The patient who relies on that signal — who does not seek private alternatives because the public system has presented itself as the responsible party — and who then discovers that the constitutional hole means the signal was never backed by an enforceable obligation — that patient is in Joshua DeShaney's position. The state intervened. The state failed. The court held that the failure was not a constitutional violation. The patient bore the cost.

Town of Castle Rock v. Gonzales

DeShaney was confirmed and extended in 2005. Jessica Gonzales had a restraining order against her estranged husband. He violated the order by taking their three daughters — Leslie, Katheryn, and Rebecca, ages seven, nine, and ten — without permission. She called the police repeatedly over the course of an evening, reporting the violation. The police did not act. Her husband appeared at the police station that night and opened fire. He was killed in the exchange. The three girls were found dead in his truck. He had killed them earlier in the evening.

Jessica Gonzales sued, arguing that the restraining order — which under Colorado law the police were required to enforce — created a property interest protected by the due process clause. The Supreme Court held seven to two that it did not. The police's failure to enforce a mandatory restraining order, resulting in the deaths of three children the order was designed to protect, was not a constitutional violation.

The constitutional hole is not a gap in the system. It is a holding of the Supreme Court. It has been affirmed twice in landmark cases involving the deaths of children. It is the foundation on which the healthcare system — with all its programs, all its coverage expansions, all its regulatory apparatus — rests. Every reform built on top of it is a favor. The floor has not been built.

What building the floor requires

The floor requires a constitutional amendment or a Supreme Court reversal. Neither is politically available in the current moment. This is the honest answer and the book owes it to the reader.

What is politically available is the construction of the programs, the precedents, and the political conditions that make the amendment or the reversal possible when the conditions shift — and conditions always shift. The ACA was enacted in a political moment that did not exist ten years before it passed and did not survive ten years after. The next window will open at a moment that cannot be precisely predicted and must be prepared for.

Every constitution in the world that built the floor did so after a period in which the argument had been made, the evidence had accumulated, and the political conditions had arrived that made the decision possible. Bismarck's Germany had the argument before it had the law. Britain had Beveridge before it had Bevan. Taiwan had decades of evidence from other countries before it had the political moment to act. The argument is in this book. The evidence is in the system's thirty-year trajectory — the rural hospital closures, the nurse departures, the physician burnout, the insulin rationing, the three daughters in the truck. The political conditions are not yet sufficient. They are forming. The fiscal crisis accelerates them. The moment will arrive.

When it does the argument must be made whole and available. The floor must be named precisely — not as the expansion of an existing program but as the constitutional recognition of what the state owes, structurally and without discretion, to every person within its jurisdiction who needs care. The DeShaney hole must be named as what it is: not a technicality of constitutional interpretation but the specific legal mechanism by which the civilization maintains the extraction apparatus at the expense of the patient at the end of the chain.

The Objectivist objection

The argument for a constitutional floor faces a serious objection from the Objectivist tradition, and the manuscript owes the reader an explicit engagement with it. The objection is not new. It was made forcefully in 1962 by Ayn Rand, addressing physicians who were resisting the King-Anderson bill that would become Medicare. Doctors, Rand argued, should refuse to accept any obligation beyond their voluntary exchange with patients who can pay. Healthcare in this framing is a normal market and should be defended as such. Any obligation imposed by a collective on an individual physician — any duty owed by the state to the citizen that requires the physician's participation — is illegitimate. The doctor is a trader, not a servant. Rand insisted this position was the consequence of a complete philosophical system she called Objectivism, grounded in specific claims about metaphysics, epistemology, and ethics, and she rejected the libertarian label firmly. The political position, in her view, could not be separated from the philosophical foundations that produced it.

Two decades later, in 1982, Leonard Peikoff — Rand's designated philosophical heir and the leading systematic exponent of Objectivism after her death — updated the argument with material that would prove uncomfortably prescient. The DRG system was being introduced. Peikoff predicted that diagnosis-related groups would produce exactly what they have produced: a system in which the physician's judgment is overridden by administrative categories, in which the quality of care declines as the categories proliferate, in which physicians retire earlier than they planned because the work no longer permits the practice of medicine, and in which costs rise rather than fall because the categories generate new forms of gaming and capture. Peikoff was right about every prediction.

The Objectivist argument has force. It is also incomplete in a way that the past sixty-three years have made unmissable. The framework treats healthcare as if it were a normal market transaction. Doctors offer services, patients buy them, both parties enter freely, the market clears, everyone benefits. This framework has been demolished — not by socialist theorists but by mainstream economics. Kenneth Arrow's 1963 paper, published one year after Rand's speech, established that healthcare violates every assumption a normal market requires. The patient cannot judge the quality of the service because medical knowledge is too specialized. The patient cannot rationally consider price during an emergency because the need is not deferrable. The patient often cannot survive without the service, which means the seller has a monopoly power that the buyer cannot refuse. Insurance creates moral hazard that breaks normal price discipline. Externalities are pervasive — one person's untreated tuberculosis is everyone's problem.

This is why every developed country in the world has reached the conclusion that healthcare cannot be organized as a normal market. The countries that have done it well — through some combination of public insurance, public provision, regulated private delivery, and the constitutional floor — have produced longer life expectancy and lower per-capita costs than the United States, which has resisted the conclusion the longest. The Objectivist position survives as a philosophical claim about the relationship between the individual and the state. It does not survive contact with the data about what produces health outcomes. Sixty-three years after Rand made the case, the country that most closely approximated her vision produces health outcomes worse than any other developed country at twice the cost.

There is something the Objectivist argument gets right and the floor argument must honor. Peikoff's prediction about DRGs was correct. The administrative capture of physician judgment is a real harm, and a constitutional floor that simply expanded the current administrative apparatus would extend that harm rather than correct it. The floor that this book argues for is not a larger version of what already exists. It is a different structure entirely — one that protects physician judgment, that pays for outcomes rather than for the gaming of categories, that recognizes the alchemy of clinical care as the work that medicine actually is. The Objectivist critique of bureaucratic medicine is correct. The Objectivist alternative to bureaucratic medicine — the unregulated market grounded in the philosophical claim that the state owes no duty to the citizen — is not the only alternative. The constitutional floor properly designed, with physician judgment protected and dignity preserved on both sides of the encounter, is another.

The argument from this book is not that Rand and Peikoff were wrong about everything. It is that they were right about the dangers of state capture of medicine and wrong about the only alternative being the rejection of any state duty toward the patient. The two errors cancel each other out in current American practice, which has produced the worst features of both: extensive state involvement that captures physician judgment without providing the floor, combined with market structures that extract rents without delivering care. The country has built the worst-case version of both arguments and called it healthcare.

The floor as the recognition of what was always true

The constitutional floor is not a gift from the state to the patient. It is the acknowledgment of what was always already true — that the person who needs care is a person, that their need does not create a market relationship, that the civilization that can provide the care and chooses not to is making a decision about whose life matters and whose does not.

The DeShaney decision called that decision constitutional. The healthcare system built its extraction apparatus on top of the decision. The law as it stands is wrong. Not technically wrong — it is the considered holding of the Supreme Court of the United States, carefully reasoned, clearly stated. It is wrong in the sense that every law that has ever been overturned or amended was wrong: because it produces outcomes that no honest accounting of what a civilization owes its members can justify.

The ninety-seven-year-old at the window. The diabetic man watching himself disappear. Alec Smith, dead at twenty-six from insulin he could not afford. Robert in Kentucky, his vascular damage accumulating during the authorization delay. The nurse who came to heal and is being required to harm. The rural hospital that served its community and was destroyed by the financial apparatus of the system it operated within. All of them are falling through the same hole. The hole is constitutional. The hole was put there deliberately. The hole can be filled — has been filled, by every other wealthy democracy that decided the patient at the end of the chain was who the system is for.

The rebuild begins with naming the hole. You cannot fill what you cannot see.

PART III

Rebuild Before Collapse

7

The Prevention Trap

Part Two was the moral argument. The system is wrong before it is expensive — wrong in its treatment of the person as a set of symptoms, wrong in its failure to see the person behind the presentation, wrong at the constitutional foundation that makes every program built on top of it provisional. Part Three is the arithmetic. The moral failure of the American system is matched only by its financial absurdity: it has engineered the most expensive possible way to produce the worst outcomes among wealthy nations. What follows is the specific clinical and economic evidence for what a different decision would cost, what it would produce, and how every country that has made that decision has benefited from it.

In 1971 James Heckman was a young economist at Columbia University beginning the work that would eventually win him the Nobel Prize. The question he was trying to answer was deceptively simple: when, in a human life, does investment produce the highest return?

The answer, documented across decades of research and replicated across countries and contexts, is this: the earlier the investment, the higher the return. The dollar spent on a child in the first three years of life produces returns — in educational attainment, employment, health outcomes, reduced criminal justice involvement, reduced public expenditure — that dwarf the returns on the same dollar spent on that child at age ten, at age twenty, or at age forty when the preventable condition has become the unmanageable one.

The Heckman Curve is not a theoretical proposition. It is the empirical finding of one of the most rigorous bodies of research in economics. It has been confirmed in studies of early childhood programs across the United States, Canada, Jamaica, and Sweden. The Perry Preschool Project, the Abecedarian Project, the Nurse-Family Partnership — each produced the same finding from different angles and different populations: the upstream investment produces returns that the downstream intervention cannot match because the downstream intervention is addressing consequences that the upstream investment would have prevented.

The American healthcare system does not fund the upstream investment. It funds the downstream intervention. Not because the Heckman Curve is unknown or disputed. Because the financial apparatus of the system is organized around a specific structural impossibility: the entity that would bear the cost of the upstream investment is never the entity that captures the return. This is the prevention trap.

How the trap works

The prevention trap is not primarily a medical phenomenon. It is a financial one. It operates through a specific mismatch between the timing of costs and the timing of benefits, combined with the fragmentation of the system that makes the mismatch permanent.

Consider a forty-year-old woman with prediabetes. Her fasting glucose is elevated but below the threshold for a Type 2 diabetes diagnosis. The clinical evidence is unambiguous: intensive lifestyle intervention at this stage prevents or substantially delays the onset of Type 2 diabetes in fifty-eight percent of cases. The intervention costs approximately four hundred dollars per person per year. The insurance company covering her this year will not fund the intervention. Not because the evidence is in dispute. Because the financial logic of the system does not support it. She may change jobs next year and leave the plan. The diabetes she develops in year eight, if untreated, will generate thirty thousand dollars in annual treatment costs — but the entity paying those costs may not be the entity that would have paid for the four-hundred-dollar prevention today. The prevention is a cost. The diabetes is a revenue stream. The insurance company that funds the prevention is subsidizing a future competitor's cost avoidance.

This is not cynicism. It is the financial logic of a fragmented, multi-payer, employment-linked insurance system applied to a chronic disease with a fifteen-year trajectory. The same logic operates across every major chronic disease category. The entity bearing the upstream cost never captures the downstream return. So the upstream investment is not made. The downstream cost arrives. It is managed — expensively, inadequately, at the stage where management is most difficult and least effective — and recorded as a new clinical event, untethered in any accounting from the upstream decision that produced it.

The billing code problem

The prevention trap is compounded by a billing apparatus that has no language for prevention. The fee-for-service billing system reimburses clinical encounters. The visit. The procedure. The test. The prescription. It cannot code the conversation that prevented the crisis. The primary care physician who spends twenty minutes discussing dietary changes, sleep hygiene, stress management, and medication adherence with a prediabetic patient has generated no billable procedure. The billing system has no mechanism to capture it. The physician who sees forty patients a day cannot afford to spend twenty minutes on prevention with each of them, because twenty minutes of prevention generates approximately the same reimbursement as six minutes of symptom management, which is to say almost nothing.

The community health worker who visits a recently discharged heart failure patient, checks their medication compliance, identifies that they have not been able to afford their low-sodium diet and connects them with a food assistance program — that visit costs forty-five dollars and prevents, with documented reliability, a thirty-thousand-dollar readmission within thirty days. The forty-five-dollar visit is not billable under most insurance contracts. The thirty-thousand-dollar readmission is fully billable. The system funds the readmission and not the visit.

The school-based mental health counselor who identifies a child's depression at age eleven, before it has become the school dropout at fifteen, the substance use disorder at nineteen, the hospitalization at twenty-three — that intervention is not a healthcare expenditure in the current billing apparatus. It is an educational expenditure, funded by school budgets that are cut when property tax revenues decline in the communities where the intervention is most needed. The system does not connect the counselor's budget to the hospitalization it prevented, because the system has no mechanism for making that connection. The hospitalization is revenue. The counselor is overhead.

The prevention trap and mental health

Nowhere is the prevention trap more devastatingly expressed than in mental health. Mental illness typically has its onset in adolescence and early adulthood. The median age of onset for anxiety disorders is eleven. For mood disorders, thirteen. For substance use disorders, fifteen. For psychotic disorders, the first episode typically occurs between fifteen and twenty-five. These are the documented epidemiology of the conditions that produce the highest long-term costs in the system.

Early intervention in mental illness changes trajectories. The research on first-episode psychosis programs is among the most compelling in the psychiatric literature: intensive coordinated care delivered in the months immediately following the first psychotic episode reduces hospitalization, improves functional recovery, and changes the long-term course of the illness in ways that years of subsequent treatment cannot replicate. The window for this intervention is narrow — measured in months, not years. After the window closes, the trajectory is harder to alter.

The system does not fund this intervention adequately. Not because the evidence is disputed. Because the billing apparatus has no adequate reimbursement code for the intensive coordinated care that first-episode programs provide — the case management, the family support, the vocational rehabilitation, the supported housing, the sustained clinical relationship that the evidence requires. The psychiatric hospitalization that follows the untreated first episode is fully billable. The program that would have prevented the hospitalization is funded through grants and state contracts that are chronically inadequate and the first target of budget cuts when fiscal conditions tighten.

For thirty-four years I ran a psychiatric nonprofit serving people with serious mental illness — people for whom the prevention window had long since closed, for whom the trajectory had been determined by decades of inadequate treatment and inadequate support. I watched staff provide extraordinary care within resources that were never adequate. I watched the reimbursement rates decline in real terms every year. I watched the population we served grow more complex as every other system — housing, criminal justice, family support — continued to disinvest in the upstream conditions that produced the people arriving at our doors. The people we served were not the casualties of their illnesses alone. They were the casualties of a system that had failed to intervene at the points where intervention would have changed their trajectories, and that then resourced the management of the consequences at the minimum level the law required and the budget permitted.

Non-adherence as a feature, not a failure

The prevention trap intersects with the non-adherence problem in a way the system is constitutionally incapable of addressing. Non-adherence — the patient who does not take their medication, who misses follow-up appointments, who does not make the dietary and lifestyle changes the treatment requires — is the single largest driver of preventable healthcare cost in the American system. The system treats non-adherence as the patient's failure. It documents it, notes it in the chart, and waits for the crisis that was always coming.

The clinical reality is different. Non-adherence is not primarily a compliance problem. It is a feature of the disease. The diabetic patient who has lost the physiological signal of satiety — whose leptin resistance and disrupted gut-brain signaling have removed the feedback mechanism that tells a person when to stop eating — cannot rely on their own body's signals to guide their dietary management. The patient with serious mental illness who stops their antipsychotic medication because they feel better is demonstrating the insight impairment that is a symptom of the illness, not a character flaw. The patient with heart failure who gains three pounds of fluid over three days and does not recognize it as a warning sign was never taught to recognize it — because the discharge from the hospitalization was rushed, the follow-up appointment was six weeks away, and the community health worker visit that would have caught the fluid retention was not billable.

A system designed to address non-adherence as a feature of the disease would build anticipatory monitoring into the treatment plan from the first encounter. It would identify, for each patient and each condition, the predictable points of non-adherence and create the clinical contact, the peer support, the practical assistance, and the medication management that address those points before they produce the crisis. Every one of these interventions is cheaper than the hospitalization it prevents. None of them is adequately funded by the current billing apparatus. The prevention trap does not only fail to prevent disease. It fails to prevent the complications of disease that the system is nominally treating. It produces the expensive crisis, then funds the management of the crisis, then produces the next crisis. The wheel turns. The cost accumulates. The patient deteriorates. The system calls this care.

The financing solution

The prevention trap has a financing solution. It is not complicated. It requires a single structural change: the entity that bears the cost of the upstream investment must be the same entity that captures the downstream return. This is the financial argument for a single-payer system or a global budget model. Not the ideological argument — the argument about what healthcare means and who deserves it. The arithmetic argument. When the same entity is responsible for the patient's health across their entire lifespan, the investment in prevention is financially rational because the return accrues to the same balance sheet as the cost.

Medicare is the partial proof of concept. Because Medicare bears the long-term cost of unmanaged chronic disease in the elderly population, Medicare has a financial incentive to fund upstream management that private insurers covering the same patient from age twenty-five to sixty-five do not have. The prevention trap is fully closed only when the entity covering the patient bears the consequences of their health outcomes across their entire life. A universal coverage system — single-payer or tightly regulated multi-payer on the German or Taiwanese model — creates this alignment structurally. The prevention trap is a product of fragmentation. The rebuild closes the trap by ending the fragmentation.

The most expensive self-devouring machine

Step back from the clinical detail and look at the whole. The United States spends more on healthcare per capita than any other nation on earth. It employs the most highly trained clinical workforce in the world. It produces the majority of the world's biomedical research. Its hospitals contain the most advanced technology medicine has ever deployed. Its pharmaceutical industry has produced treatments that have transformed the course of diseases that were once death sentences.

And it has organized all of this capacity around a system that systematically destroys the conditions for its own effectiveness. It eliminates the time that clinical wisdom requires. It defunds the prevention that would reduce the acute burden. It burns out the workforce whose moral reserves sustain the gap between what is reimbursed and what is required. It closes the rural hospitals that serve the communities most dependent on them. It produces the complications it was built to prevent, then charges for managing those complications, then produces the next complications. It is not failing. It is succeeding at the wrong thing, with extraordinary efficiency, at maximum cost.

This is what the scarcity orientation looks like when it is institutionalized at civilizational scale. Not the individual who hoards against mortality. The civilization that has organized its most important human service around extraction rather than care, around the billing code rather than the person, around the quarterly earnings report rather than the patient's trajectory across a life. Every layer of the apparatus consuming what it was built to protect. The insurance company consuming the premium. The hospital consuming the community's trust. The pharmaceutical company consuming the scientific commons that made the drug possible. The political system consuming the democratic mandate that gave it authority to act.

The American healthcare system is not a failure of intelligence or technology or resources. It is what extraordinary intelligence, technology, and resources look like when organized around the wrong purpose — the most sophisticated self-devouring machine in the history of organized medicine, too elegant to collapse quickly, too entrenched to reform easily, and too expensive to sustain indefinitely. The smartest and most technologically advanced nation has built the most expensive system that produces among the worst outcomes in the wealthy world. That is not an accident. It is the design. And the design can be changed — but only by a civilization that is willing to look at what it has built and name it for what it is.

8

The Disease Map

The ten most expensive disease categories in the American healthcare system account for the majority of the four-and-a-half-trillion-dollar annual expenditure. They are not evenly distributed across the population. They are concentrated in specific demographic groups, in specific geographies, and at specific points in the disease's natural history — points that, in almost every case, could have been reached later or avoided entirely with upstream investment that the system systematically refuses to make.

What follows is a map — the specific location in each disease's natural history where the system currently spends its money, where the evidence says the spending should occur, and what the financial and human cost of the gap between those two points has been. The map is the clinical evidence for the rebuild. Not the policy argument. The specific, disease-by-disease, point-by-point demonstration that the prevention trap is not a theoretical construct. It is the operating reality of the American healthcare system, expressed in the conditions that are destroying it from the inside.

Diabetes — $327 billion annually

Type 2 diabetes is the American healthcare system's most expensive preventable disease. Three hundred and twenty-seven billion dollars annually is spent managing a condition that develops over years, announces itself clearly at the prediabetes stage, and responds reliably to intervention at that stage in the majority of cases.

The prediabetes population in the United States is approximately ninety-six million people. Of those, approximately eighty-four percent do not know they have it. Of the sixteen percent who do, a small fraction receive the structured lifestyle intervention that prevents progression. The CDC's National Diabetes Prevention Program — the evidence-based intervention with documented efficacy — reaches less than five percent of the eligible population.

The reason is familiar. The intervention requires time, sustained engagement, dietary support, regular monitoring, and motivational counseling. The billing apparatus does not adequately fund any of these. The insurance company covering the prediabetic patient will not bear the cost of her diabetes in fifteen years — she will be on Medicare, on a different plan, or uninsured. The prevention is a cost. The diabetes is someone else's revenue.

The complications arrive on schedule. The amputation costs eighty thousand dollars. The dialysis costs ninety thousand dollars per year. The cardiovascular event costs forty to a hundred thousand dollars for the acute intervention. The system funds all of these — fully, promptly, without prior authorization delay — because the billing codes are unambiguous and the acute intervention is what the system was built to provide. It will not fund the four-hundred-dollar annual prevention program.

Non-adherence in diabetes compounds everything. The patient who has lost the physiological satiety signal cannot rely on their body's feedback. The patient whose blood glucose is not catastrophically elevated does not feel acutely ill — the damage is invisible and accumulated. The dietary changes required conflict with the food environment of the communities where diabetes is most prevalent. Non-adherence in diabetes is not primarily the patient's failure to comply with instructions. It is the system's failure to design treatment around the actual conditions of the patient's life.

Cardiovascular disease — $250 billion annually

Heart disease remains the leading cause of death in the United

States. The majority of this expenditure occurs in the acute phase — the myocardial infarction, the stroke, the heart failure hospitalization, the cardiac procedure. The upstream story is well established. Hypertension, the primary modifiable risk factor, affects approximately one hundred and twenty million Americans. Of those, only about one in four has it adequately controlled. The medications that control hypertension are inexpensive — generic antihypertensives cost pennies per day. The barrier is not pharmacological. It is the system's failure to identify, monitor, and support adherence in the population at risk.

The vascular damage accumulates invisibly. The event arrives — sudden, acute, billing-code-clear. The cath lab activation, the stent, the cardiac rehabilitation. All of it funded promptly and completely. None of it connected in any accounting to the years of inadequately controlled hypertension that produced the event.

Mental health and substance use disorders — $280 billion annually, and undercounted

The two hundred and eighty billion dollar figure is almost certainly a substantial undercount. It captures direct mental health and substance use treatment expenditures. It does not capture the cardiovascular disease driven by untreated depression. The diabetes complications driven by psychiatric comorbidity. The criminal justice costs of untreated mental illness and addiction. The emergency room visits that are the de facto mental health system for people who have no other access. The true cost of undertreated mental illness and substance use disorders — when all downstream consequences are included — is conservatively estimated at over a trillion dollars annually.

The treatment gap is enormous. Approximately half of Americans with a diagnosable mental health condition in any given year receive no treatment. The gap is widest in rural areas and in low-income populations where the barriers of cost, transportation, insurance coverage, and stigma are highest. The system's primary response to untreated mental illness is custodial: the emergency room, the inpatient psychiatric unit, the jail or prison that has become the de facto mental health institution for the most severely ill. The emergency room visit for a psychiatric crisis costs approximately two thousand dollars and addresses nothing underlying. The inpatient admission at fifteen to thirty thousand dollars provides stabilization and discharge back to the same conditions that produced the crisis.

For thirty-four years I ran a psychiatric nonprofit serving people with serious mental illness — people for whom the prevention window had long since closed, for whom the trajectory had been determined by decades of inadequate treatment and inadequate support. The people we served were not the casualties of their illnesses alone. They were the casualties of a system that had failed to intervene at the points where intervention would have changed their trajectories, and that then resourced the management of the consequences at the minimum level the law required and the budget permitted.

Obesity — $173 billion annually, and upstream of everything

Obesity is not primarily a disease of individual choice. It is the downstream consequence of multiple upstream failures operating simultaneously on a biological system not designed for the nutritional environment of the modern food industry. Leptin resistance disrupts the satiety signaling that would otherwise regulate food intake. Disrupted sleep dysregulates the hormones that control appetite and metabolism. The chronic stress of economic insecurity promotes fat storage and metabolic dysfunction. The food environment of low-income communities provides abundant access to ultra-processed calories and restricted access to whole foods.

The GLP-1 medications that have demonstrated remarkable efficacy for both obesity and its cardiovascular and metabolic complications are among the most significant pharmacological developments in recent decades. They are being denied by prior authorization, priced out of reach for the patients who need them most, and their coverage is being actively restricted by insurance companies. The patients who cannot access these medications will develop the diabetes, the cardiovascular disease, the metabolic syndrome that the medications would have prevented — at costs that dwarf the medication's price. Obesity is upstream of diabetes. It is upstream of cardiovascular disease. The system that refuses to treat obesity is not avoiding a cost. It is deferring multiple costs into the future while they compound with interest.

Alzheimer's and dementia — $321 billion annually

Three hundred and twenty-one billion dollars annually, the majority borne by families rather than by the healthcare system — the informal care that does not appear in the financial accounting but consumes the lives of the people providing it. There is no disease-modifying treatment for the majority of Alzheimer's cases. What the system can do, and largely does not, is address the care needs of the person with dementia and their family across the disease's trajectory — not merely in the acute phases that generate hospitalizations but in the sustained, daily reality of living with progressive cognitive decline. The caregiver providing forty hours a week of unpaid care. The person with early dementia who could benefit from structured programs that extend function and dignity across the disease course. The system funds the hospitalizations. It does not fund the sustained care that makes the hospitalizations less frequent or the disease course less devastating. The prevention trap here takes its most complete form: no entity in the current system captures the financial return on investing in that sustained care, because the primary return is borne by the unpaid family caregiver — who does not appear in any budget, who cannot bill for the hours, and whose exhaustion and breakdown will eventually generate their own healthcare costs that the system will also fail to prevent.

Cancer — $200 billion annually

Cancer is the disease category where the prevention and early detection argument is clearest and the system's failure to act on it is most consequential. Cervical cancer is virtually eliminable through vaccination and screening. The HPV vaccine, if universally administered at the recommended age, prevents the majority of cervical cancers. Colorectal cancer, detected early through colonoscopy or stool-based testing, has a five-year survival rate above ninety percent. Detected late, it falls below fifteen percent. The barriers are familiar: cost, access, transportation, the primary care relationship that would identify screening gaps — all of the upstream investments the system does not make. The late-stage cancer treatment that results from screening failure costs hundreds of thousands of dollars per patient. The screening that would have caught it early costs a few hundred.

The common thread

Across every disease category in this map, the same pattern appears. The system spends the most money at the point of intervention where money is least effective — the acute event, the late-stage complication, the crisis that could have been prevented. It spends the least money at the point where money is most effective — the early detection, the lifestyle intervention, the medication that prevents the complication, the clinical relationship that addresses non-adherence before it produces the hospitalization.

The gap between where the money is spent and where it should be spent is not a clinical judgment. It is a financial one, produced by the structural mismatch already described: the entity bearing the upstream cost never captures the downstream return. Fix the financing. Close the fragmentation. Align the incentives with the evidence. The disease map changes. The system that treats diabetes at the prediabetes stage rather than the amputation stage will spend less and produce better outcomes. This is not complicated medicine. It is what every other wealthy healthcare system has already learned. The American system has not learned it not because the knowledge is unavailable but because the financial apparatus that would have to change belongs to the most politically powerful industries in the country.

9

Prevention Is Not Billable

The American healthcare system cannot prevent what it did not cause. The diseases driving the system's financial collapse — diabetes, cardiovascular disease, serious mental illness, substance use disorders, obesity, Alzheimer's, cancer — do not begin in the clinic. They begin in the food desert and the unstable home and the school without a counselor and the community that has been systematically disinvested for decades. The clinic is where the disease presents. The disease was produced elsewhere, over years or decades, by conditions the healthcare system has no instrument to address and no billing code to capture.

A billing code for the diabetes diagnosis. No billing code for the food desert that made the diet impossible. A billing code for the hypertension medication. No billing code for the housing instability that makes the medication schedule unmanageable. A billing code for the psychiatric hospitalization. No billing code for the adverse childhood experience that made the psychiatric crisis predictable twenty years before it happened. The system bills for the disease it was too late to prevent. It cannot bill for the prevention it was never designed to provide. And so it does not provide it.

The rebuild that this book argues for is not primarily a healthcare reform. It is a civilizational one. The prevention of the diseases that are destroying the system requires investments that exist entirely outside the healthcare system's institutional boundaries — in food policy, housing policy, early childhood investment, education, community infrastructure, and the built environment.

The social determinants are not social

The phrase "social determinants of health" has been in the public health vocabulary for decades. It suggests that the factors outside the clinic are somehow softer, less medical, less urgently clinical than the factors inside it. They are primary causes. The ACE study — the Adverse Childhood Experiences study, following more than seventeen thousand patients — established that childhood trauma is dose-dependently associated with every major expensive adult disease category. The person with four or more adverse childhood experiences has a seven-fold increased risk of alcoholism, a six-fold increased risk of depression, a twelve-fold increased risk of suicide attempt, and dramatically elevated risk of heart disease, cancer, chronic lung disease, and liver disease. These are among the strongest predictive relationships in the epidemiological literature. The adverse childhood experience is a primary cause of the expensive adult disease. Not a background variable. A clinical cause, as direct in its mechanism as a pathogen.

Food

You cannot treat obesity in a food desert. The patient who leaves the clinic with a dietary counseling sheet and returns to a neighborhood with no grocery store within three miles, two fast food restaurants within walking distance, and a dollar store where the cheapest calories are the most processed — that patient has received a prescription they cannot fill. Not because they lack motivation. Because the environment makes the prescription impossible. The healthcare system cannot change the food environment. Only food policy can. But the healthcare system that pretends the food environment does not exist — that hands the dietary counseling sheet and records the counseling as provided — is participating in the performance of prevention rather than its provision.

Early childhood

The brain architecture laid down in the first three years of life determines the stress response system, the immune function, the metabolic set point, the capacity for emotional regulation — all of which are upstream causes of the most expensive adult diseases. The child whose early environment is characterized by instability, neglect, poverty, and chronic stress develops a stress response system that is hyperactivated, difficult to down-regulate, and associated across the lifespan with elevated inflammatory markers, metabolic disruption, and the psychiatric and cardiovascular conditions that dominate the expensive end of the disease map. This is neuroscience, not social policy. The healthcare system addresses none of it. Early childhood investment is not a healthcare expenditure in the current apparatus. The return on this investment is primarily captured by the healthcare system decades later, in the reduced prevalence of the expensive adult diseases that early adversity produces. The healthcare system does not make the investment. It manages the consequences.

Housing

Housing is health. Unstable housing is independently associated with worse outcomes in virtually every chronic disease category. The Housing First model — providing permanent supportive housing to chronically homeless individuals — produces better health outcomes and lower total system costs than the shelter-and-treatment model. The permanent supportive housing unit that ends the cycle of homelessness costs approximately ten to twenty-five thousand dollars per person per year. The emergency room visits and hospitalizations that characterize the healthcare utilization of chronically homeless individuals cost multiples of this amount. The healthcare system funds the emergency room visits. It does not fund the housing. Not because the evidence is in dispute. Because the housing is not a healthcare expenditure in the current apparatus.

Education, mental health, and community

Education is the single strongest predictor of health outcomes across the lifespan — stronger than income, stronger than access to healthcare. The school that is funded by local property taxes in a poor district, with overcrowded classrooms, no school nurse, no counselor — that school is a health intervention that fails before the child reaches adolescence. Mental health conditions, untreated, are upstream causes of virtually every expensive physical disease category. Depression is an independent risk factor for cardiovascular disease with outcomes comparable in magnitude to smoking. Untreated anxiety drives cortisol dysregulation, immune suppression, and metabolic disruption. The system that cuts mental health funding first in every budget cycle is not saving money. It is deferring costs into every other budget line and paying compound interest on the deferral in human suffering that never appears in the financial accounting.

Loneliness is a health risk equivalent to smoking fifteen cigarettes a day. The community organizations, the faith institutions, the neighborhood infrastructure that produces social connection are prevention at a scale no clinical intervention can match. They are not healthcare expenditures. They are what gets defunded when local governments face budget pressure. The rural community that lost its hospital also lost the community gathering place the hospital represented. None of this is in the healthcare budget. All of it determines what the healthcare budget will spend.

The comprehensive case

The healthcare system cannot prevent what the conditions of life produce. The conditions of life are determined by decisions made in food policy, housing policy, education policy, environmental policy, economic policy, community investment, and the built environment. The healthcare system has no institutional voice in most of these decisions. The industries that make these decisions have no accountability for the healthcare costs their decisions produce.

A comprehensive prevention strategy is not an expanded healthcare budget. It is the alignment of every policy domain with the recognition that the conditions of life determine health — and that the civilization that allows those conditions to deteriorate while funding the expensive management of the consequences is making the same choice the extraction apparatus makes in every individual billing encounter: deferring the upstream cost because the entity bearing it is not the entity that will capture the return. The entity that will capture the return — or pay the price for failing to capture it — is the civilization itself. Somebody always decides. The question is whether the decision is made deliberately, with the full accounting of what the conditions of life produce, or by default, with the costs deferred to the future and the bill paid in the suffering that prevention would have spared.

10

What Taiwan Decided in Two Years

In 1994 Taiwan had a healthcare problem that looked, in several important respects, like the American healthcare problem of today. Forty percent of the population was uninsured. Coverage was fragmented across multiple government programs, each with different benefits, different contribution structures, and large gaps between them. The poor, the elderly, the self-employed, and the geographically isolated fell through those gaps with the predictable consequences: delayed care, advanced disease at presentation, medical bankruptcy, preventable death.

In 1994 the National Health Insurance Act was passed. In 1995 the new system was operational. By the end of 1995 Taiwan had achieved near-universal coverage: ninety-two percent of the population enrolled in the first year, rising to ninety-nine percent within a decade. The administrative cost of the new system was six percent of total healthcare spending. The United States administrative cost at the time was approximately thirty percent. Within a decade, health outcomes were improving across every major category. The total cost of the system stabilized at approximately six percent of GDP. The United States today spends eighteen percent. Taiwan covers everyone. The United States does not. Two years from political decision to operational universal system.

What Taiwan actually built

Taiwan's National Health Insurance is a single-payer system. It is not a government-run healthcare system. The hospitals and clinics remain largely private. The physicians remain largely independent practitioners. The government does not employ the doctors or own the hospitals. It pays them — at negotiated rates, through a single administrative channel, without the multiple-payer administrative overhead that consumes thirty cents of every American healthcare dollar.

Every resident of Taiwan is enrolled. The contribution is income-based — individuals, employers, and the government all contribute proportionally. There is no premium that prices the low-income patient out of coverage. There is no deductible that defers the first-dollar cost onto the patient who most needs care. There is a modest copay for office visits — approximately five to ten US dollars — that reduces unnecessary utilization without creating the financial barrier that drives the American uninsured to defer care until the condition is acute. The administrative simplicity is not incidental. It is the source of the cost savings that make universal coverage financially viable. One set of claim forms. One payment schedule. One administrative channel. The army of billing staff that American hospitals employ to navigate four hundred different insurance plans does not exist. The prior authorization department does not exist. The PBM extracting the rebate does not exist. The money that is not spent on administrative overhead is spent on care.

The transition that the American debate says is impossible

The standard American objection to the Taiwan comparison is familiar. Taiwan is smaller. Taiwan is more culturally homogeneous. The American healthcare industry is too large, too politically powerful, too deeply embedded in the economy to be transformed on any comparable timeline. Each of these objections contains partial truth and fundamental misdirection.

The scale objection is precisely backwards. A larger single payer has more negotiating leverage with drug manufacturers and hospital systems. The Medicare program, covering sixty-five million Americans, already demonstrates this — Medicare's administrative costs and reimbursement efficiency substantially exceed those of private insurers covering far smaller populations.

The cultural homogeneity objection mistakes political will for cultural consensus. Taiwan's transition was achieved through political decision, not cultural uniformity. The coalition that passed the National Health Insurance Act was the coalition of the insufficiently covered: the self-employed, the agricultural workers, the low-income elderly, the dependents who fell between the existing programs' gaps. The American equivalent of that coalition exists. It is the coalition of the uninsured and underinsured working class that the extraction apparatus has spent decades preventing from recognizing its common interest.

The entrenchment objection is the most serious. The American private health insurance industry, the pharmaceutical industry, and the hospital consolidation economy represent trillions of dollars in entrenched capital and political investment. Their resistance to a Taiwan-style transition would be formidable. It would not be insurmountable. The Canadian physicians who went on strike against the introduction of Medicare in 1962 are now among the most vocal supporters of the system. The British medical establishment that bitterly opposed the creation of the NHS in 1948 became one of its most committed institutional defenders. Entrenchment is real. It is not permanent. It yields to the combination of fiscal crisis, political will, and the intellectual clarity that names the system for what it is.

The administrative savings calculation

The United States spends approximately thirty-four percent of its total healthcare expenditure on administrative costs — billing, coding, prior authorization, claims processing, marketing, executive compensation. Taiwan spends six percent. Germany spends less than ten percent. Canada spends approximately twelve percent. The difference — twenty to twenty-five cents per dollar on a four-and-a-half-trillion-dollar system — is between eight hundred billion and one trillion dollars annually. This is the money currently consumed by the extraction apparatus. Moving it from administrative overhead to the coverage of the uninsured is not a tax increase. It is a reallocation.

What the transition requires

The Taiwan transition was made possible by three conditions that the United States does not currently possess and must build. The first is political will — the specific combination of legislative majority, executive commitment, and public pressure that makes structural reform possible. The second is administrative infrastructure — the enrollment systems, the payment systems, the data systems that a single-payer transition requires. Medicare already provides much of this. The expansion of Medicare to cover all Americans would build on existing administrative capacity rather than creating new institutions from nothing. The third is the managed transition for the workers currently employed in the extraction apparatus. The insurance industry, the billing and coding industry, the prior authorization infrastructure employ millions of Americans whose jobs would be displaced. This is a real cost. It is not an argument against the transition. It is an argument for designing the transition carefully.

The proof of concept is not theoretical. Every wealthy democracy that has achieved universal coverage has proven that the technical and financial barriers to the transition are surmountable. Germany proved it in 1883. Britain proved it in 1948. Canada proved it in 1966. Australia proved it in 1975. Each transition was contested. Each faced the opposition of entrenched interests. Each system now produces better outcomes at lower cost than the American system. The American exceptionalism argument — that the United States is uniquely unsuited to universal coverage — is the argument of the industries that benefit from the extraction apparatus. It is not a factual claim. It is a political strategy. Somebody always decides. Taiwan decided in two years. The question for the United States is not whether the decision is possible. It is when the conditions will produce the political will to make it.

11

The System That Sees the Person

Every rebuilt system begins with a question. The question determines the design. The wrong question produces the wrong system, however efficiently designed, however well-funded, however earnestly administered. The American healthcare system was built around the wrong question. The question it answers with extraordinary sophistication is: how do we code, bill, and reimburse the clinical encounter? The question it has never been designed to answer is: what does this person need to be well? These are not the same question. The first produces a billing apparatus. The second produces a healthcare system. The rebuild requires starting with the second question and designing everything else around the answer.

The answer is not uniform. It depends on who the person is, what their history is, what the conditions of their life are, what they value, what they are capable of, and what their specific disease at this specific moment in their specific life requires. This is what clinical medicine has always known and what the billing apparatus has always been designed to ignore. What follows are the design principles of a system organized around the person rather than the presentation.

Design principle one: Time

The most important resource in clinical medicine is time. Not technology. Not pharmaceuticals. Not facilities. Time — the clinical time in which the person across the desk can stop presenting the edited version and start presenting the actual one. The time in which the symptom can be traced to its source rather than coded at its surface. The time in which the non-adherence can be understood rather than documented. The time in which the treatment plan can be designed around the conditions of the actual life rather than the idealized patient the fifteen-minute slot was built for.

A system built around the whole person restores time by changing what gets paid for. Not time itself — time cannot be billed as a commodity without creating perverse incentives. What gets paid for is the outcome that time produces: the patient who does not return to the emergency room because the follow-up call caught the deterioration. The patient whose depression was addressed before it became the cardiac event. Capitation models, global budgets, and accountable care organizations with genuine risk-sharing all create financial incentives for the time investment that prevents the expensive downstream event. The specific staffing requirement follows: the primary care physician who carries a panel of two thousand patients and sees forty patients a day cannot provide the time that person-centered medicine requires. The rebuilt system requires panels of twelve to fifteen hundred, appointment slots of twenty to thirty minutes for complex patients, and the team structure — nurse practitioners, pharmacists, community health workers, behavioral health specialists embedded in primary care — that distributes the work across the people best positioned to provide it.

Design principle two: Continuity

The whole person becomes visible through continuity. The first encounter produces the edited version. The fifth encounter, with the same clinician, in a relationship that has accumulated enough trust to make the editing unnecessary, produces something closer to the actual person. Continuity is what the current system systematically destroys. The insurance plan that changes with employment changes the primary care relationship. The narrow network that excludes the established physician changes it. The single-payer system that covers the patient regardless of employment eliminates the insurance transition that destroys the primary care relationship. The entity accountable for the patient's health across their lifespan has the incentive to maintain the continuity that person-centered medicine requires.

Design principle three: The full person in the record

The electronic health record as currently designed is a billing document that also contains some clinical information. The billing apparatus required fields are there. The person's own account of their illness, their preferences, their living situation, their support network, their history of adverse experiences, the goals they have for their life that the treatment should serve — these appear inconsistently, in free-text fields that are not searchable, in notes that are not transmitted between providers. The rebuilt record captures the person as the primary subject of clinical attention rather than the presenting symptoms as the primary subject of billing. The advance care document specifying preferences at the end of life, accessible to every clinician, maintained and updated across the lifespan. The social circumstances that determine whether the treatment plan is actually executable. This is the documented content of records maintained by primary care practices in countries that have built person-centered care into their systems — the Netherlands, Denmark, the United Kingdom — where the primary care record is genuinely longitudinal, genuinely personal, and genuinely useful.

Design principle four: Prevention as the primary obligation

The rebuilt system reverses the current system's temporal logic. The current system is organized around the acute event. Prevention is a secondary activity funded from what remains after the acute system is resourced. The rebuilt system makes prevention the primary obligation and acute care the failure mode. The community health worker embedded in the primary care practice who does the home visit that catches the fluid retention before the readmission. The behavioral health specialist integrated into primary care who addresses the depression before it drives the cardiac event. The pharmacist who reviews the medication list and identifies the interaction before it produces the emergency room visit. None of these roles is adequately funded in the current system. All of them are cheaper than what they prevent. The rebuilt system funds them because the system accountable for outcomes across the lifespan has the financial incentive to fund the upstream intervention that prevents the downstream cost.

Design principle five: The constitutional floor

The system that sees the person cannot be built on sand. The constitutional hole — the Supreme Court's holding that the government has no affirmative obligation to provide care — means that every program, every coverage expansion, every prevention investment built on top of it is subject to political revision, budget cutting, and the managed care organization's quarterly review. The person-centered system requires the constitutional floor. Not as a philosophical preference but as a structural requirement: the system designed to see the whole person across their lifespan cannot function if the coverage that makes that longitudinal relationship possible can be withdrawn by administrative decision. The German Basic Law makes this commitment for the German person. The Canadian Constitution Act makes it for the Canadian person. The American constitution does not yet make it for the American person. The rebuild requires that it does.

Design principle six: The AI instrument

Augmented intelligence is the specific technology that makes person-centered care scalable. Not because it replaces the clinician. Because it makes visible what the current system cannot see. The patient whose HbA1c has been drifting upward for three years without a medication adjustment. The patient whose depression screening has been positive at every visit without generating a referral. The patient whose medication list contains an interaction that has never been flagged. The patient whose housing situation has changed in ways that make the treatment plan no longer executable. Augmented intelligence applied to the longitudinal record — without ideological stake, tasked explicitly with whether the patient is receiving the care the evidence says they should be receiving — produces the accountability mechanism that makes person-centered care enforceable. Not to replace the physician's judgment. To support it. To flag the drift before it becomes the crisis.

What the rebuilt system produces

The patient in the rebuilt system has a primary care relationship that has lasted long enough for the editing to stop. The clinician knows their history from the accumulated experience of the longitudinal relationship. The treatment plan was designed around the conditions of their actual life. The non-adherence was anticipated and addressed before it produced the crisis. The depression was identified and treated before it drove the cardiac event. The prediabetes was caught and managed before it became the amputation.

When the acute event comes — because acute events come regardless of prevention — the system responds without the prior authorization delay, without the narrow network exclusion, without the chargemaster price that bears no relationship to cost. The event is managed as what it is: a clinical problem requiring a clinical response, funded by the system as a whole rather than extracted from the individual encounter.

At the end of life, the preferences that were documented across the longitudinal relationship are honored. The conversation that happened at sixty-five has been updated at seventy-five and again at eighty. The clinician who will be present at the end knows what this person values. The system does not override those preferences with the acute intervention that maximizes the billing encounter and minimizes the human dignity.

The person was seen. The whole person. Across the lifespan. As the full human being they always were. That is the rebuilt system. That is what the constitutional floor makes possible. That is what the extraction apparatus made impossible for the four and a half trillion dollars it consumed. Somebody decided that the extraction apparatus was what the system would be. Somebody can decide the person-centered system instead.

12

What Other Countries Decided

Taiwan decided in two years. But Taiwan is not the only proof of concept, and it is not the most instructive one for every dimension of the American problem. Different countries solved different parts of the problem. Different countries started from different basements and arrived at different systems. What they share is the decision — made at a specific historical moment, against real opposition, by leaders who named the extraction apparatus for what it was and chose to replace it. Each country's story teaches something specific that the Taiwan story alone cannot teach. Together they constitute the evidence that the American exceptionalism argument is not a factual claim. It is a political strategy. The facts are the outcomes. And the outcomes, across every wealthy democracy that made the decision, are the same: better health at lower cost, with the patient at the center rather than the billing code.

Germany: the conservative case

The first thing to understand about Germany's healthcare system is who built it. Not a socialist government. Not a progressive reformer. Otto von Bismarck — the Iron Chancellor, the architect of Prussian conservatism, the man who unified Germany through blood and iron — enacted the world's first statutory health insurance in 1883. His logic was explicitly not humanitarian. It was strategic: the working class without a floor was a working class available for revolution. The Bismarck lesson for the American debate is precise: universal coverage is not inherently a left-wing proposition. It is a stability proposition. The society that allows the conditions of working-class life to deteriorate beyond a threshold produces political instability that is more costly than the floor would have been. The American political leadership that has spent forty years opposing universal coverage as socialism has missed the lesson that the father of modern conservatism understood in 1883.

Germany's system today is a regulated multi-payer model — approximately ninety not-for-profit sickness funds competing for members on the basis of service quality, but not on the basis of coverage. The essential benefit package is standardized. No fund can deny coverage or charge differential premiums based on health status. The result: universal coverage, administrative costs below ten percent, out-of-pocket costs capped at two percent of annual income, drug prices negotiated by the government. The system has operated continuously for one hundred and forty years through two world wars, hyperinflation, division, and reunification. What Germany teaches: universal coverage does not require a single payer. It requires the regulatory commitment that makes the market serve the patient. The American multi-payer system with German regulation would produce German outcomes.

Japan: the cost argument

Japan spends eleven percent of GDP on healthcare. The United States spends eighteen percent. Japan covers everyone. The United States does not. Japan's life expectancy is among the highest in the world. The United States ranks approximately forty-sixth globally, below every other wealthy democracy. Japan's social insurance model sets the fee schedule through government negotiation, caps patient cost-sharing, and negotiates pharmaceutical prices every two years based on comparative effectiveness. The drug that offers no improvement over existing treatments receives no price premium. The result is universal coverage at substantially lower cost without rationing, without inferior technology, without limitations on physician freedom. What Japan teaches: the cost of the American system is not the cost of healthcare. It is the cost of the extraction apparatus layered on top of it. Every country that has eliminated that apparatus spends substantially less and covers everyone more completely.

Canada: the proximity argument

Canada is the comparison the American healthcare debate cannot avoid and consistently misrepresents. Same continent. Shared border. Similar cultural baseline. Universal coverage. Better outcomes on most measures. Lower cost. Canada's Medicare — enacted federally in 1966, building on provincial programs operating since the 1940s — is a single-payer system at the provincial level. The essential benefit package is defined federally. Variations in wait times for elective procedures are real and are consistently exaggerated by American critics. The Canadian patient who waits twelve weeks for an elective knee replacement has a better outcome than the American patient who cannot afford the procedure at all. Canada's universal coverage system was built against the fierce opposition of the Canadian Medical Association and political forces that made exactly the same arguments that American opponents make today. It was built anyway. It has produced, over sixty years, a healthier population at lower cost than the American system that was not built.

Australia: the hybrid argument

Australia's Medicare covers every Australian for essential medical services, hospital care, and pharmaceutical costs above a threshold. Private insurance supplements but does not replace the public system — approximately half of Australians hold private supplemental coverage for amenities, shorter wait times for elective procedures in private hospitals, and services not covered by Medicare. The hybrid model addresses the American fear that universal coverage eliminates choice. In Australia it does not. The patient who wants the private room and the private surgeon can purchase the supplemental coverage. The patient who cannot receives the essential care that Medicare guarantees. The floor is universal. The ceiling is private. Total healthcare expenditure:

approximately ten percent of GDP. Universal coverage. Life expectancy among the highest in the world. What Australia teaches: the floor does not require the elimination of the private ceiling. It requires the commitment that every person has the floor, regardless of their ability to purchase the ceiling.

The Nordic model: the integration argument

The Nordic countries — Sweden, Norway, Denmark, Finland — spend between ten and twelve percent of GDP on healthcare and produce the best population health outcomes in the world on most measures. But the Nordic lesson is not primarily about healthcare. It is about the floor as an integrated commitment. Healthcare in the Nordic countries is one component of a comprehensive floor that includes universal early childhood care, quality public education through university level, robust unemployment insurance, universal elder care, and housing policy that prevents the homelessness that drives emergency room utilization in the United States. The prevention trap is substantially closed not because the Nordic healthcare system is better designed than the German or Taiwanese system, but because the conditions of life that produce the expensive diseases are addressed across every policy domain simultaneously. What the Nordic model teaches is the argument of Chapter 9 confirmed at civilizational scale: the diseases that drive healthcare cost are substantially preventable upstream, in the conditions of life, rather than managed downstream, in the clinic. The countries that built the floor across the conditions of life are healthier and spend less. The connection is causal, not coincidental.

The common decision

Germany 1883. Britain 1948. Canada 1966. Australia 1984. Taiwan 1995. Different systems. Different political moments. Different institutional arrangements. The same decision underneath all of them: the healthcare system is for the patient, the floor belongs to every person by right of being a person, and the state's obligation to deliver it is not discretionary.

Each decision was made against opposition. Each opposition made the same arguments that American opponents make today: too expensive, too radical, a threat to quality, a step toward socialism, an infringement on individual freedom. Each argument was wrong. Not wrong in the abstract — wrong in the specific, documented, measurable sense that the systems built against that opposition produce better outcomes at lower cost than the system the opposition was protecting.

The United States has not yet made this decision. Not because the decision is impossible. Because the political conditions that would make it politically irresistible have not yet arrived. They are arriving. The fiscal crisis accelerates them. The visible failure of the rural hospital closure, the nurse departure, the physician burnout, the insulin rationing — these accelerate them. The moment will come. The question is whether the argument is clear and available when it does. This book is the argument. The decision is the work.

Epilogue

Epilogue: Rebuild

The findings are not ambiguous.

The American healthcare system spends more per person than any other in the world and leaves more people uncovered, sicker, and more financially destroyed by the cost of their care than any comparable nation. The gap between what it costs and what it produces is not a market inefficiency. It is the designed output of an apparatus built to extract value from the clinical encounter rather than deliver care. The extraction is legal. It is politically protected. It has been maintained through the most sophisticated lobbying infrastructure in American political history. And it is consuming itself — depleting the clinical workforce, closing the rural hospitals, rationing the insulin, producing the complications it was built to manage and managing them at maximum cost.

The major hurdles are not clinical or financial. The money is already in the system. The clinical knowledge exists. The models from other countries are documented and available. The hurdles are political: the financing apparatus that converts the industries' profits into the political outcomes that protect those profits, the revolving door that makes the regulators the regulated, and the misdirection that has kept the system's primary victims voting for the representatives who maintain it.

What other countries teach is that these hurdles are not permanent. Germany crossed them in 1883. Britain in 1948. Canada in 1966. Taiwan in two years, from forty percent uninsured to universal coverage. Each transition was made against opposition that used identical arguments to the ones deployed in the United States today. Each system now produces better outcomes at lower cost. The political conditions that made those transitions possible were not planned. They arrived — fiscal crisis, visible failure, the coalition of the harmed finally recognizing its common interest. They are arriving here.

How to proceed is the question the evidence answers: build the floor. Not as a program that can be cut, not as a policy that can be repealed, but as the constitutional recognition that every person within this country's jurisdiction has the right to the care their life requires. Fund the upstream investment — the prevention, the early intervention, the person-centered primary care — that addresses the disease before it becomes the crisis. Align the financial incentives with the patient's health across their lifespan rather than with the extraction from each billing encounter. Eliminate the administrative apparatus that consumes thirty cents of every premium dollar and redirect it to care.

None of this waits for the constitutional amendment. It begins with the clarity that names the system for what it is. The physician who names the moral injury. The nurse who refuses to accept the unsafe staffing ratio as simply how things are. The patient who insists the prior authorization denial is a system failure. The citizen who looks at Alec Smith and asks not what he could have done differently but who decided the insulin would cost three hundred and fifty dollars.

Ultimately this is a problem of will and values. The political leader, the institutional administrator, the board member, the citizen — each faces the same choice the evidence has made unavoidable: whether to value humanity over profitability, the person over the billing code, the floor over the extraction. Without healthy citizens

— without the basic floor of food, housing, and healthcare that makes a life genuinely livable — the nation is hollow. And the leaders of a hollow nation are leading what, exactly? Not a civilization. Not a people. A revenue stream with a flag. The floor is not charity toward the weak. It is the condition of everything the nation claims to be. You cannot have a strong country built on sick, indebted, undertreated people. You cannot have a democracy built on citizens too exhausted by survival to participate in it. The choice is not between profit and idealism. It is between a nation that works and one that does not. Every other wealthy democracy made that choice. The evidence of what it produces is available. The will to make it is the only thing missing.

The decision was made. It can be made differently.
The window is open. The argument is complete. It is time to decide and act for the floor.

Sources and Acknowledged Cases

Named cases referenced in this book:

Alec Smith (1991–2017): Type 1 diabetic, died June 27, 2017, after rationing insulin. Account drawn from extensive reporting in the Minneapolis Star Tribune, NPR, and congressional testimony by his mother Nicole Smith-Holt.

Robert Allen (Kentucky): Type 2 diabetic with vascular complications, account drawn from Kentucky Public Health Association documentation and patient advocacy reporting on rural hospital closures and insulin access.

Trishaun Holland: Mental health crisis case referenced in reporting on emergency department mental health holds, drawn from health journalism investigations of psychiatric bed shortages and emergency department boarding.

Rural hospital closures: 146 closures and 432 at-risk facilities cited from the Cecil G. Sheps Center for Health Services Research, University of North Carolina (2023–2024 data) and American Hospital Association reports.

Healthcare spending data ($4.5 trillion, 18% of GDP): Centers for Medicare and Medicaid Services, National Health Expenditure data (2023–2025).

Medical debt and bankruptcy data: Kaiser Family Foundation, Consumer Financial Protection Bureau, and American Journal of Public Health peer-reviewed research on medical debt as cause of bankruptcy.

Comparative international data: OECD Health Statistics 2024–2025, World Bank Health Data, and Commonwealth Fund Mirror, Mirror reports on international health system comparison.

Heckman Curve and early childhood ROI: James J. Heckman, Nobel laureate economist, University of Chicago, multiple peer-reviewed publications on early intervention return on investment.

Kenneth Arrow, "Uncertainty and the Welfare Economics of Medical Care," American Economic Review, December 1963 — the foundational analysis of healthcare market failures.

DeShaney v. Winnebago County Department of Social Services, 489 U.S. 189 (1989), and Town of Castle Rock v. Gonzales, 545 U.S. 748 (2005): U.S. Supreme Court decisions establishing the absence of affirmative constitutional duty of the state to protect.

Ayn Rand, "Medicine: The Death of a Profession," speech delivered at Ford Hall Forum, 1962, collected in Philosophy: Who Needs It (1982). Leonard Peikoff, "Medicine: The Death of a Profession" lectures and writings on DRGs, available through the Ayn Rand Institute.

International healthcare system histories: Taiwan (1995 single-payer transition under William Hsiao consultancy); Germany (Bismarck 1883 sickness fund legislation); Britain (Beveridge Report 1942, NHS Act 1946, NHS operational 1948); Canada (Tommy Douglas, Saskatchewan 1962, federal Medical Care Act 1966).

Where statistical figures or specific claims appear without inline attribution, they are drawn from the sources above or from the broader peer-reviewed health services research literature. The argument of this book rests on the empirical record. The empirical record is publicly available.

Index

Page references are to the printed edition.

Index

Also by Ravinder Nath Bhalla, MD

WISDOM IN PSYCHIATRY

Wisdom in Psychiatry: Understanding Begins Healing

Nietzsche: A Guided Tour

The Money Book Nobody Gave You

Before the Birth of Hope and Despair

THE ABUNDANCE SERIES

Book One *Abundance: Beyond Scarcity and Self-Devouring Cycles*

Book Two *The Twin Minds: Choosing Abundance over Scarcity*

Book Three *Red Lines Rising: Governing AI While We Still Can*

Book Four *The Abundance Dispatch: Letters to Power*

Book Five *Building Abundance: What We Ought to Create*

Book Six *The Constitution: Floor Missing*

Book Seven *The Abundance Life: A Guide from Birth to Posterity*

About the Author

Ravinder Nath Bhalla, MD, is a board-certified psychiatrist (adult and child) with forty years of clinical practice and thirty-four years as medical director of a nonprofit serving underprivileged populations across a wide age range. He led a team of psychiatrists and consulted to local school districts.

He is the author of thirteen books, including the seven-volume Abundance Series (ABUNDANCE; The Two Minds: Choosing Abundance Over Scarcity; Red Lines Rising; Abundance Dispatch; The Constitution: The Floor Missing; Building Abundance; The Abundance Life), Wisdom in Psychiatry: Understanding Begins Healing, Nietzsche: A Guided Tour — A Path Through His Works (two-volume box set), Wealth, Mind and Meaning: The Money Book Nobody Gave You, What Does It Mean to Be Human In the Age of Robots and Augmented Intelligence, and The World Constitution: What We Owe to Our Children Present and Future. A fourteenth book, Before the Birth of Hope and Despair: On Life, Death, and Heritage, is forthcoming.

His work addresses civilization's defining challenge: the contest between abundance and scarcity orientations at every scale, from the individual life to the constitutional floor to the civilizational architecture now being shaped by augmented intelligence. He is the creator of the Abundance Index, a live tool at ravibhallamd.-com/abundance-index that calculates the cost of ending world hunger and extreme poverty as a fraction of global military spending.

He maintains a small private practice and writes from the

United States. The full body of work is available at ravibhallamd.com.

Made in the USA
Monee, IL
13 September 2026

62981876R00066